Signe Brunnstrom

Physical Therapy Pioneer, Master Clinician and Humanitarian

Jay Schleichkorn, PhD, PT

SLACK Incorporated, 6900 Grove Road, Thorofare, New Jersey 08086

SLACK International Book Distributors

In Europe, the Middle East and Africa:
John Wiley & Sons Limited
Baffins Lane
Chichester, West Sussex P019 1UD
England

In Canada:
McAinsh and Company
2760 Old Leslie Street
Willowdale, Ontario M2K 2X5

In Australia and New Zealand:
MacLennan & Petty Pty Limited
P.O. Box 425
Artarmon, N.S.W. 2064
Australia

In Japan:
Igaku-Shoin, Ltd.
Tokyo International P.O. Box 5063
1-28-36 Hongo, Bunkyo-Ku
Tokyo 113
Japan

In Asia and India:
PG Publishing Pte Limited.
36 West Coast Road, #02-02
Singapore 0512

Foreign Translation Agent

John Scott & Company
International Publishers' Agency
417-A Pickering Road
Phoenixville, PA 19460
Fax: 215-988-0185

Publisher: Harry C. Benson
Managing Editor: Lynn C. Borders
Editor: Cheryl D. Willoughby
Designer: Susan Hermansen
Production Manager: David Murphy

Printed in the United States of America

Library of Congress Catalog Card Number: 89-42994

ISBN: 1-55642-127-3

Published by: SLACK Incorporated
6900 Grove Road
Thorofare, NJ 08086

Last digit is print number: 10 9 8 7 6 5 4 3 2 1

To My Wife
Marianne

Table of Contents

Acknowledgments

This author wishes to acknowledge the cooperation and assistance given by many people in developing this biography. In particular, appreciation is extended to Signe Brunnstrom's immediate family; her sisters, Elsa Brunnstrom Diehl of Lund, Sweden and Ingegerd Brunnstrom Westerlund of Stockholm; as well as her niece, Elsa Diehl of Westport, Connecticut. Without their sharing of letters, papers, photographs, documents and books, Signe's story could not have been told.

I am very grateful to the many close friends and colleagues whose lives were touched by Signe Brunnstrom. In a most cordial manner, they were quick to share and contribute information. They include Mary Eleanor Brown, Mary Callahan, Anthony DeRosa, Ruth Dickinson, Sam Feitelberg, Mary Flickinger, Jack Hofkosh, Geneva Johnson, Althea Jones, Jeanne LaVigne, L. Don Lehmkuhl, Kerstin Lundbladh, Stuart MacRoberts, Elfriede Prins, Kathy Sawner, Sarah Semans, Lucy Gore Stead, Francis Tappan, Robert Teckemeyer, and G. Gordon Williamson. They were among more than 100 people (listed in Appendix III) who took the time to respond to my requests for personal views, specific information and anecdotes.

Thanks to all.

Foreword

Anna Signe Sophia Brunnstrom—a meteor that will forever glow—has enlightened and enlivened the world of physical therapy. The Brunnstrom legacy is told by Jay Schleichkorn in this gripping biography of the woman who personifies the alluring comprehensiveness of physical therapy. Signe Brunnstrom has expanded the neurophysiologic underpinnings of human movement through her methods of clinical research and application. But more than that, her impact is upon all health professions as she works out her effective methods and sees them into print amidst the intricacies she encounters in her daily life and work.

This spell-binding account of adventures brings Signe from Sweden and takes her to and from faraway places. For sources, Dr. Schleichkorn went to Sweden and to numerous colleagues and students, including myself. I see whirlwind Signe Brunnstrom as an animated statue of liberty freeing us for greater and greater clinical practice and research.

I remember Signe as a vibrant woman full of energy, robust health, goodness, goodwill, friendliness, good cheer, diligence, enormous motivation, high intelligence, and scientific fervor to find the truth, in order to help her patients, her students, her colleagues, her friends, and her profession.

Athletically inclined, this friendly woman lived a physically active life to the fullest. She thought hard, read and studied hard, did her paintings, gardened, and built parts of her country place, solved problems, traveled, and worked zestfully in overwhelmingly complex conditions.

For me, Signe Brunnstrom epitomizes the best in physical therapy. She reflects the highest ethical conduct. The Brunnstrom ways of operating are creative. She invented her work schedules to accommodate her singleness of purpose, the search for treatment methods that work. The Brunnstrom way of daily life and work illustrates the power of discipline and integrity to build confidence, a necessary ingredient in any profession. Her methods abound in lessons for practicing physical therapy successfully. I revelled in her insistence on learning on oneself. She palpated muscles on herself that few can find. I was a ''learner'' rather than a pupil or a student. She read in several languages and dredged from the most abstruse material the stuff out of which she created her neurophysiologic approaches to her patients. It is with joy that I recall the joyful responses from patients, students, colleagues, audiences—and an exuberant Signe!

There is a storybook quality about the harrowing circumstances surrounding Signe's beloved country retreat. Dr. Schleichkorn has successfully interwoven these tragic episodes among the concentrated work periods. Despite the misfortunes, this ebullient woman played herself out in an overfull life span leaving us with invaluable insights and procedures.

This biographer records for those who have not yet known Signe the life and works of this great physical therapist. A practiced writer of biographical and other works, he enhances his subject with a cursive style, copious quotes, Signe diary entries, and a profusion of photographs and illustrations. His fine work reflects monumental industry, appreciation for detail, compassion, and an enviable sense of history.

This biography is an important part of the history of physical and occupational therapy, medicine, and rehabilitation. It is also a sociologic document showing ways to function in a society in which highly motivated individuals may expend and fulfill their energies on ill segments of the population, dogs, horses, and many other aspects of nature—as did Signe.

Jay Schleichkorn gives us an enjoyable book about the evolution of a physical therapist from a young ''Director of Gymnastics'' from Sweden excelling in calisthenics to a master clinician who leads us down new avenues into the mysteries of human motion.

An inspiring adventure awaits the reader of the Signe Brunnstrom adventures within.

Mary Eleanor Brown

Preface

Sweden has a notable historical record for producing outstanding individuals who have served mankind, particularly in the fields of art, science, engineering, diplomacy and medicine. While a list of the most famous might be quite long, among those persons easily recognizable are Bergman, Bernadotte, Bjoerling, Garbo, Hammarskjold, Lind, Ling, Nilsson, Nobel and Strindberg. Each made unique and lasting contributions to Sweden and the world.

To any list of Swedish-born notables one should add the name of Signe Brunnstrom. She was an educator, clinician, researcher, author and humanitarian. Her accomplishments have been shared primarily with the professions of physical therapy and occupational therapy and those related to physical rehabilitation. Her contributions have affected and benefited innumerable people—and will continue to do so—especially for those patients who have been exposed to the "Brunnstrom approach."

How Signe Brunnstrom influenced the lives of many professional personnel as well as their patients can best be described by chronologically tracing her life and career of more than 90 years. The twilight of her years was spent in a nursing center, dependent on nursing staff to meet all of her needs. How ironic that such a dynamic, enthusiastic and energetic woman, who spent her life demonstrating and teaching others how to rehabilitate the disabled, should find herself totally incapacitated. For all the professional personnel who were touched by this most remarkable woman, it is best to remember her as she was. Signe Brunnstrom has a special place in the history of rehabilitation. Lest we forget the important role she played in physical therapy and rehabilitation, this publication was prepared after intensive historical research and with the cooperation and input of many people.

Perhaps, somewhere in the health field, some readers will attempt to emulate the commitment, dedication and service to their profession and patients so overwhelmingly demonstrated by Signe Brunnstrom, to the benefit of mankind.

Jay Schleichkorn, PhD, PT

Chapter One

The Early Years

"Long before World War II, I had been frustrated when called upon to treat patients with hemiplegia, but it was not until after the war that I really began to tackle the problems of these patients. The clinics at that time were comparatively well-oriented to war injuries, such as amputees and paraplegics, but stroke patients were badly neglected a 'polio approach' was universally used." With those words, written by Signe Brunnstrom, the very foundation of her enthusiastic approach to bring about change in the rehabilitation of the hemiplegic patient is established.

Where and how did it all begin? What were the major influences in the life of this intelligent yet shy Swedish individual? What brought her international recognition and loneliness at the same time? People who were fortunate enough to know Signe found her unforgettable. Those who never had the opportunity to be in her presence should be made aware of her influence and dedication to professional service.

In describing the life of Signe, an appropriate place to start is in the mid-1800's. The Brunnstrom family has deep roots in Sweden. On August 14, 1860, a son was born to Fabian Wilhelm Rudolf Brunnstrom and Christina Elisabeth Engstrom in Vastra Ramlosa, Helsingborg, Sweden. He was named Magnus Rudolf Mauritz Edvin Brunnstrom and was to be known as Edvin. The family eventually would include a daughter Hanna and two other sons, Fabian and Leopold.

Although the Brunnstroms owned a farm in Pilshult, Edvin was not destined to be a farmer. He attended school in Halmstad where he met his wife-to-be, Hedwig Sofia Lidman.

Edvin was born into a family steeped in the military tradition and accordingly, he followed a military career, as did his brother, his father, his grandfather and his grandfather's brother. He served with an infantry regiment in North Scania in 1878 and passed an officers examination to be a lieutenant in 1880. With a junior rank in the army between 1880 and 1889, his income was not quite sufficient to take on the responsibilities of married life. A promotion to captain in 1890 helped to make the difference. In 1894, after a long engagement Edvin married Hedwig, who by then had graduated from the Teacher Training College in Stockholm.

A year after the marriage, the Brunnstrom's first child, Elsa Sofia Kristina, was born on December 21, 1895. Three years later, when a second child was due, an interesting situation occurred that was often humorously discussed by the family.

Imagine you are going to a gala party—all dressed up in your finest and very comfortable in a warm taxi—when suddenly you are stopped and ordered to get out. The demand to vacate your vehicle does not come from a criminal or an officer of the law but from a middle-aged woman, dressed in a cape and carrying a small black leather bag. She is a midwife! She needs transportation to get to her patient, a mother ready to deliver a baby. You and your companion do not complain about missing the anticipated revelry of the evening and quickly comply with her request. That was the situation in Stockholm on December 31, 1897, New Year's Eve of 1898. In those days a midwife had the right to commandeer a vehicle to undertake her important duties.

At Karlberg Castle, the Swedish Military Academy, Hedwig Brunnstrom was ready to deliver her second child. As an officer, Edvin used the only phone in the academy to call the midwife. Shortly after midnight, January 1, 1898, even before the midwife arrived, the Brunnstroms had another-daughter. She was named Anna Signe Sofia. Such was the beginning of the life of one individual who was to make major contributions to the field of physical therapy, rehabilitation and care of the disabled.

In 1905, the Brunnstroms had their third daughter, Ingegerd Sofia, born August 2. (Is it possible Captain Brunnstrom was hoping for a son who would eventually follow the military tradition? Little did he know that one day it would be Signe who would carry on the family tradition.)

While one would think the life of a military officer has certain advantages, it was not easy for the Brunnstroms. In 1908, Edvin was a major with the regiment at Kalman. He also worked for five summers at the general's Staff Topographic Division. Being a career military man meant that Edvin was often required to spend time away from home tending to his duties. This also involved relocating to different areas when he received a new assignment. The Brunnstrom family moved often to such places as Ljunghbyhed, Ronneby, Jonkoping and Eksjo.

While this could have caused great disruption of the Brunnstrom children's education, it must be remembered that Hedwig Sofia Brunnstrom was well-educated. She was a teacher of French, German and English. In addition to all of her motherly duties, Hedwig assumed the responsibility for the education of her daughters. Her ability to do so was accepted by school authorities after an unannounced visit to the home. They observed a lesson and were most impressed with the educational level of the children. Hedwig taught the children until 1909 when Edvin was placed in command of a regiment and stationed in Eksjo. There, Signe and Elsa attended school and easily kept up with the curriculum. Education was a major part of their life but they still found time to be very involved in gymnastics, skiing, ice-skating and horseback riding. They also took part in the "girl guides" movement and participated in nature activities, care of animals and learning about Swedish history. This was the time, Signe's strong love for animals and interest in sporting activities were crystallized. Those interests were to last a lifetime.

In December 1984, I met with Signe's younger sister, Ingegerd Brunnstrom-Westerlund, in Stockholm. She related an incident that demonstrated Signe's concern for horses on a winter day in Eksjo. Feeling sympathetic for the animals, Signe enlisted a group of friends to put snow back on the cleared streets in order to make it easier on the horse's hoofs!

Life in Eksjo was soon disturbed. It was a time of great national concern as World War I started on July 28, 1914, when Austria-Hungary declared war on Serbia. Although the war was in a distant land, there was anxiety in Sweden. Ingegerd recalled how soldiers of her father's regiment attended a church service in 1914, and how impressed they were with the danger. Throughout World War I, Sweden maintained its neutrality, but the Swedish people faced hardships with shortages of food, certain clothing and commodities. Elsa and Signe often found themselves waiting on long lines to purchase rationed fish or other food. Many times their wait was in vain and they were unsuccessful in bringing home needed supplies.

Signe was now sixteen years old and it was time to further her education. Being athletically inclined and interested in sports, Signe planned to enter physical education. She majored in science at Uppsala College where she studied physics, chemistry, mathematics, and biology, as well as religion, philosophy, French, English, history, geography and gymnastics. Almost a straight "A" student, she continued her studies in physical education and physiotherapy at the Royal Gymnastic Institute in Stockholm. Excerpts from a letter of June 4, 1935, written while living in New York City, described her educational pursuits between 1915 and 1919:

> The educational plan in Sweden differs considerably from the American high school/college/university plan. The secondary school and college lead up to a final examination called the 'Student-examen', or Bachelor's

> degree. It is equivalent to the German 'Maturitetsexamen' and to the French 'Baccalaureat'. I passed this 'Student-examen' in Uppsala, Sweden in 1917. I have been in a position to compare our Swedish studies with American colleges and I have found that in most respects a "Student-examen" is equivalent to a B.S. or B.A., though American universities do not allow more than two years of college credit for our Swedish College (Gymnasium).
>
> After graduation from Uppsala College, I entered Kungl. Gymnastiska Central-Institutet (The Royal Central Institute for Gymnastics) in Stockholm. This school is a combined Physical Education and Physiotherapy school of two years duration. I received my degree on 30 May 1919 and the title of "Gymnastikdirektor." This school has university standing and a graduate of the school is entitled to practice physiotherapy and to teach physical education in Sweden.

While at the Central Institute, Signe received the nickname of "Ensign" from her classmates because she was the tallest student in the class and a leader. Webster's dictionary defines ensign as "a badge, a symbol, or token of office or authority, a standard bearer." The Certificate of Citizenship issued to Signe Brunnstrom on November 26, 1934, indicates she was five feet ten inches in height.

At the Institute, Signe excelled in calisthenics. She was greatly influenced by the work of the renowned Swedish gymnast, Per Henrik Ling (1776–1839) whose techniques were taught at the Royal Institute. The use of Swedish Gymnastics was the foundation for much of Signe's treatment approaches with all types of disabled persons. Photographs taken in Switzerland, Greece and New York confirm how Signe applied the Ling exercises in various situations throughout her career.

Adopting Ling's work demonstrated Signe's ability to integrate scientific thinking and practical application. Edgar Bick (1968) in his *Source Book of Orthopedics* described Ling's work:

Ling developed the ancient Greek art of calisthenics to a science based upon sound anatomic and physiologic principles. He was among those who thought in terms of motions rather than muscles, and believed that the education of the locomotor system was the best way to prevent the occurrence of idiopathic deformities such as scoliosis, round shoulders, hollow back or weak feet. Ling worked intensively to perfect his methods, and succeeded in interesting not only the profession in his own country, where he founded the now famous Swedish School of Physiotherapy, but the profession in the rest of the world as well. After Ling, scientific body building by rational calisthenics became a recognized procedure not only for the weak child or adult, but, of even greater consequence, as an integral part of the plans for preventative medicine which were taking form in the schools of gymnasia of all civilized nations. (Courtesy of the New York Academy of Medicine Library)

Calisthenics played an important role in one of the first positions Signe held after graduation from the Royal Academy in 1919. She worked at a special health resort-spa in Medevi. A tradition at the facility involved all the guests taking part in a walk after breakfast. With flags, a brass band and drums leading the group, it was known as the "Porridge Parade." This was followed by outdoor morning exercises and a cross-country run led by Signe. It could be said that Signe Brunnstrom was jogging long before the activity became so popular!

Signe was also involved with an organization known as Red Star. (As a point of interest, the organization changed its name to Blue Star when the Soviets adopted the red star as their symbol). This was a group of equestriennes who were supervised and trained by military personnel to handle horses. An accomplished rider, Signe expected to be sent to Finland after the war to teach others about equestrian care. She never received the assignment but learned a lot about horses.

In 1920, Signe Brunnstrom left Sweden to establish residence in Berne, Switzerland. She joined a Norwegian physical therapist who ran a small treatment center. Through a contact with the Swiss Accident Insurance Institute, Signe was encouraged to establish her own physical therapy private practice in Lucerne. In 1921, she had a small "Sjugymnastik Institute" in the basement of the home of a Dr. Pometta at Dreilindenstrasse 12. Her reputation as a therapist grew quickly and her schedule was expanded. Signe was interested in treating disabled children and took very little money for her services. Wealthy patients who came to Lucerne as tourists were charged accordingly. Signe also saw a need to offer exercise programs to working women. She rented a gymnasium in a local school and set up evening classes. Home visits to polio patients also took a lot of time. All of these activities required moving about Lucerne so Signe obtained her first car, a Citroen (probably in 1923). For rest and relaxation, Signe maintained her interest in such outdoor activities as horseback riding, playing tennis, skiing and canoeing.

With a stronger financial position, Signe reached out to help her younger sister Ingegerd obtain an education. Signe made arrangements for Ingegerd to come to Lucerne where she spent April, 1923 through March, 1924 at the city's commercial school for girls. Signe paid for Ingegerd's board. This was just one of the many acts that demonstrated Signe's generosity and concern for helping others. Throughout her life she gave little thought to surrounding herself with luxuries and she was not materialistically-inclined. She preferred to share or give things away.

By 1925, Signe needed larger quarters and a more central location. She moved her institute to Kappelplatz number 5. (In October 1925, Margit von Schwerin, one of Signe's dear friends, gave her a photo album that depicted the clinical work in Lucerne.)

About this time, Signe obtained a working partner. It was hoped that the additional therapist would ease Signe's caseload and allow Signe to develop new areas. One of her major interests was to establish an exercise program for women factory workers. She thought that as many as fifteen to twenty women would be interested, but when a program was announced, 150 applications were received. Unfortunately, Signe's co-worker became ill and could not manage the workload. Signe had to work twice as hard to meet a demanding schedule. This was a trait that would reveal itself time and time again in Signe's future. The partnership was dissolved in 1927, and Signe decided to leave Switzerland and establish a practice in the United States.

Chapter Two

The New York Experience

Arriving in New York in 1928, Signe Brunnstrom was another individual in the big city searching for a job that would allow her to do what she most enjoyed doing—working with patients in physical therapy and teaching. According to her sister Ingegerd, the first several years in New York were quite difficult for Signe. People took advantage of her good nature. She obtained a position working in the gymnasium at the Hospital for Ruptured and Crippled on East Forty-Second Street. Her immediate supervisor was Dr. Kristieng Hansson. Work hours were long and there was little vacation time but she had the opportunity to develop her teaching skills and practice "physical therapy." With her primary training in Sweden devoted to exercise therapy, it should be noted that Signe was not exposed to the type of physical therapy curriculum offered in today's professional programs. She had an innate ability to integrate all of her knowledge and experience. This is borne out by a Swedish physical therapist, Birgit Ahnmark of Stockholm, who worked at the hospital in 1931. In May, 1985, Birgit wrote Ingegerd:

> We were 14 Scandinavians working in the physiotherapy department. There I met Signe Brunnstrom who had been working there some years. She was a leader

> and had much experience from various duties in this field. She was good looking, had fair hair and friendly brown eyes, she was capable and had travelled. For me, having recently moved to the U.S.A., it was a great help to be able to turn to her, asking for advice, which she gave freely—a generous friend. I admired her incredible patience. . . . it is with deep and happy gratitude I remember the good comrade and friend Signe Brunnstrom.

In 1929, Signe lived on the Upper West Side of Manhattan at 360 Riverside Drive. This was a tree-lined area overlooking the Hudson River that must have reminded her of some European cities. To meet her financial obligations she found a second job on as the ''physical training instructress'' in the gymnasium of the Metropolitan Life Insurance Company . There she was able to apply her ideas about working women taking part in physical education activities, similar to what she had established in Switzerland. Under her direction female employees participated in a very active health and exercise program. Metropolitan Life recognized the need for employee physical fitness long before the concept became popular in the 1970s. Sessions were held on Tuesdays and Thursdays in the late afternoon and evenings in Metropolitan's large gymnasium at One Madison Avenue. For ten a session, Signe taught calisthenics, gymnastics, posture control and served as the women's basketball and volley ball coach. Payroll records from Metropolitan indicate she made 20 dollars a week in the early years. Twenty years later, she would make 40 dollars. Times were bad for many people in New York during those years following the stock market crash on October 29, 1929 and no doubt the extra income was very important to Signe.

Signe's employment application mentions Margit Aden of 20 East 8th Street as a friend to call in case of an emergency. Ms. Adin was a physiotherapist. Margit remained a very close friend for many years.

It did not take dynamic Signe long to find other opportunities and professional activities. Besides her work at the hospital and with Metropolitan Life, she assisted in teaching some exercise classes at New York University, saw patients for a Dr. Cobb, consulted at the Institute for Crippled and Disabled (ICD) and had what may be referred to today as a ''private practice'' offering Swedish massage. She soon had several wealthy clients in the city, and one in particular was Josef Willem Mangelberg. He was a Dutch-born conductor of the London Symphony Orchestra from 1911 to 1914. In the United States, Mangelberg conducted the National Symphony, and after the merger he conducted the New York Philharmonic for nine seasons from 1921 to 1929. The Maestro and his wife always made sure Signe had tickets for concerts as she enjoyed such cultural activities. They became very close friends, and in January 1930, when Signe needed medical care, the Mangelbergs helped her. Suffering from increasing menstrual pains, Signe was recommended for surgery to remove a tumor. She was totally disenchanted with the medical services she saw and hesitated about having any surgery in New York City. The Mangelbergs insisted on Signe going to Europe for hospital care and they accompanied her to Germany. On February 22, following the surgery, Signe wrote her sister Ingegerd from Giessen, Germany. Being in top physical condition, Signe's surgery for what was referred to as a ''woman's problem'' did not restrain her activities for very long. Upon returning to New York City she went back to her strenuous work routine.

Signe's relationship with the insurance company lasted through 1953, with many interruptions for military service, lecture tours and teaching assignments, all without pay. Her sister Ingegerd emphasized the fact that ''Metro appreciated her efforts and allowed her time off.'' On August 7, 1931, payroll records show that the gymnasium was ''to be closed on days scheduled for the women while Miss Brunnstrom is absent.''

How Signe affected the lives of many of the office personnel at Metropolitan is best demonstrated by comments obtained from ''alumni'' members of the insurance firm. An article appeared in Metropolitan's Alumni Magazine in May, 1985, asking the readers to submit reminiscences about their relationship with Signe which could be included in a biographical publication. Four responses were received by Editor Peter English.

From Marian M. Oliva of New York City:

> I retired from Metropolitan Life as Secretary to the Chief Executive Officer in 1983, and had been an employee for forty-five years. At the time when I met Miss Brunnstrom in the Metropolitan gymnasium, I was a relatively new employee in the early 1940's, and took her classes after office hours—believe I went into the early 1950's.
>
> Upon our first visit to her classes my girl friend and I were concerned for different reasons. I, being at that time "too thin" was fearful of losing weight and my friend, who felt she was "too plump" was fearful she might not.
>
> When we approached Miss Brunnstrom with our concerns she assured us that the only exercise that would make us lose pounds was to "push away from the table real hard three times a day" and that was the best advice I ever got.
>
> Her classes were enjoyable, and in retrospect she was very much "ahead of the times" I find, with all the emphasis now on keeping fit. Since my retirement I have been in an exercise class at the 53rd Street YWCA here in Manhattan where we do much the same regime as Miss Brunnstrom taught.

From John R. Stevens of Cleveland Heights, Ohio

> Because of her work as a physical therapist, I was able to improve my own health through exercise. I was born as a "blue baby." An insurance man who worked for the Met brought Signe's work to my attention. I am old retired veteran from Metropolitan and I still jump rope, chin, stand on my head, etc. Signe gave me the idea like she has influenced many more.

From Muriel Mahon, June, 1985:

> I remember Signe B very well. She made me stretch many an arm or leg in the gym in the good old days and she did it with a smile and a determination that she'd see that you did it and all with a very pleasing personality. I used to think of her as the 'Greta Garbo of the physical world.'

From Margaret Mary Brown of St. Petersburg, Florida, formerly of Metropolitan's Field Management:

> I remember this fine lady very well. I had just been employed by the Company. This was my first taste of my chosen career, office work. However, I was only 16 years old, and I was full of energy of youth. The wonderful gym was a boon to me. I was a very active athlete, and the excellent calisthenic classes provided by Miss Brunnstrom were the answer to my needs. There was no unpleasant discipline, only good advice as to why it was good to participate in the classes. We also had thc benefit of excellent instruction and guidance. I particularly remember Miss Brunnstrom's caution about using machines. She advised us to seek her knowledge as to which of the machines would be beneficial for our personal requirements. The exercises I learned in that gym, so many years ago are the same that are being advocated today, and the cautions have been repeated to me over so many years, but I had a good instructor, and knew how careful one should be with the mechanical devices. Ms. Brunnstrom also introduced the theory that a machine will not do it all, and talked of diet and the need for some outdoor activity. The manner of touching one's toes and coming up slowly, one vertebrae at a time was one of this good lady's tenets, long before the fashionable health spas came into being. I never knew to where this good lady disappeared. I am glad to let her know I have

> never forgotten her. She was always genial and interested in her Metropolitan girls. Please say "Thank you," to a wonderful lady from one who is still enjoying the dividends of having been a pupil.

It is obvious that Signe's plan for Metropolitan's exercise program was well-thought-out and ahead of its time. One need only look at the number of employee exercise programs available today to recognize that Signe saw all of this in the early 1930s and 1940s, truly demonstrating her remarkable insight.

Signe was careful with her funds to the point of being frugal, for she was able to save enough money to once again help Ingegerd. From August, 1931 through June, 1932, Ingegerd attended the Prince School in Boston, majoring in economics. Signe took care of the financial arrangements. On occasional weekends in the summer, the two sisters spent time together at Cape Cod enjoying the sun, the beach and swimming.

Continuing her education was also important. In September 1931, she was admitted to Barnard College in Manhattan "on credentials satisfactory to the Acting Dean." There she registered as a "non-matriculated special student" for premed science courses. She took nine credits of chemistry and a three-credit English course. All courses were passed with a grade of "B".

She also enrolled at New York University for courses in the 1932–1933 school year. Among the courses she took were "Principles of Methodology in Physical Education and Organization", "Examination and Efficiency Tests", "Principles of Physical Education", "Educational Sociology", and "American Education: Its Past and Outlook".

In addition to her schoolwork, Signe decided to write a booklet titled, *Corrective Gymnastics in the Treatment of Poor Posture, Curvatures of the Spine and Weak Feet*. The complete double-spaced typed manuscript of 71 pages with 104 illustrations was found among her personal belongings. Signe wrote: "The purpose of this pamphlet is to serve as an aid for instructors in Corrective Gymnastics." The material kept in an old Sphinx Business Paper box included various exercises that Signe used for years, primarily in Sweden and Switzerland. The table of contents included General Principles, Examinations and Records, Nomenclature, Poor Posture, Kyphosis and Lordosis, Scoliosis, Weak Feet, Schedules and a Bibliography. Every illustration was hand-drawn and then silhouetted. The preface indicates the paper was typed in New York in 1932. Signe also had a sub-title for the pamphlet, *A Handbook of Corrective Physical Education*. Recognizing that she had only arrived in the United States four years earlier and that English was not her major language, the manuscript clearly indicated Signe's potential for creating future publications. There is no indication that the material was ever published and it remains in the musty box.

A decision was made in 1934 that becoming a physician would be too costly and time-consuming, and the plan was dropped. On June 4, 1935, Signe wrote:

> I was not in a position to study medicine, as I did not have enough money to carry me through four years of medicine. Instead, I decided to study for a Master's Degree in the Department of Physical Education, New York University. I will have completed my courses at the end of the summer session and I expect to receive my degree at the end of the summer this year.

November 26, 1934, was a very special day. At the age of 36, Signe became a citizen of the United States of America. Her naturalization took place in the Southern District of New York City. At the same time, she officially had a name change by "decree of the court" from Anna Signe Sofia Brunnstrom to Signe Brunnstrom. Her address was given as 500 Riverside Drive.

By October 1935, NYU had granted her a Master of Arts degree. Even after receiving the degree, Signe continued her education at NYU and took courses in the 1935–36 and 1938–39 school years. These courses included "Fundamentals of Body Mechanics", "Principles of Educational Psychology" and "Personality and Social Adjustment". Her transcript indicates she received a grad of "P" in all courses except one, "Analysis and Procedures in Correcting Postural Defects". For some reason she did not complete the course and it became an "automatic 'F' ".

About this time, Dr. Hansson recognized Signe's ability to teach and arranged for her to serve as an instructor in the hospital's program for physical therapists. From this period on we have correspondence from physical therapists who came to know Signe well. One such person was Emily "Sue" Fairbanks of Bradenton, Florida, who went on to be a physical therapist in the U.S. Army:

> I was a student of Signe Brunnstrom in 1935–36 when she was an instructor in Therapeutic Exercise for Dr. Hansson at the Hospital for Ruptured and Crippled. Her specialty at that time was therapeutic exercise for scoliosis and other musculoskeletal problems.

Another individual who studied at the Hospital was Harry B. Doppelt of New Windsor, New York:

> My friendship with Signe goes back to 1935 when I started as a physical therapy student at the Hospital. Signe was the first person I met in physical therapy. She was teaching and working in the gymnasium during 1935–36. I recall she had very little interest in treatment modalities. One particular time she was filling in at the clinic and had to turn to me, a student, to find out how to properly connect the electrodes of the longwave diathermy machine. Her forte was kinesiology and its therapeutic applications. I could relate to this because I already had some background in physical education and this was essentially my field of interest. Signe was keenly analytical. Exercises had to be based on the precise function of muscle groups. I became so engrossed in muscle function that I read everything I could get hold of. Signe also had a social consciousness which may have been due to her Scandinavian background. In 1936, the only way you could be licensed to practice physical therapy in New York State was to

graduate from a four year college course. A small group of PT's including Signe and myself, attempted to get the law changed. This was attempted through membership in the State, County and Municipal Workers of America. We met several times with the Union lawyer. We didn't get very far at the time because of the medical lobby, but it was an early effort to gain recognition for therapists.

In spite of an intense work and study schedule, Signe developed an interest in landscape painting. Starting with water colors, she sat for hours alongside the East River in New York City putting her impressions of the skyline on paper. This was carried over to the period she spent in California where rooftops and tropical plants caught her eye. Only nine such paintings are in existence and all demonstrate a unique understanding of combining colors with contemporary subjects.

Signe, with her creative mind, had to share her observations and information with others and what better way than through writing and publishing. In late 1934, only six years after arriving in this country, she prepared her first article, written in English, *Faulty Weight Bearing: With Special Reference to Position of Thigh and Foot*. It was published in the Physiotherapy Review, (Vol. 15, No. 3, 1935). This was the forerunner of the 22 articles, several chapters in books, numerous abstracts, book reviews, three voluminous research reports, and three major books that make up the legacy of professional literature authored by Signe Brunnstrom. And that does not include grant proposals and five films! Harry Doppelt recalls meeting with Signe from time to time in those early years:

> For a while she was living in Tudor City, close to the hospital. Later she lived in Greenwich Village and also had a summer place, the converted "chicken coop" in Carmel. She eventually built a more elaborate place close to the coop. It was sometime in 1937 that Signe invited me and a friend (later my wife) to a summer cottage in Darien. We went for a swim in a nearby lake

and it started to rain. I headed back to the cottage because it was getting cold. The rain didn't phase Signe. She dove into the water and had her swim, cold or not. I envied this vigorous woman!

But that was Signe. She loved the outdoors and physical activities. She divided her time between several jobs, receiving her education, seeing private patients, enjoying the summer cottage, horseback riding, gardening, and serving her profession. At the same time her analytical mind questioned the concepts of movement and therapeutic exercise.

On October 3, 1936, Signe applied for a passport through the passport agency in New York City. In the summer of 1937, she was off to Sweden for a visit with her family. She also managed to present some lectures at the Seraphim Hospital in Sweden. As a result of the visit, she tried to establish an exchange program with the hospital and the Institute for Crippled and Disabled. Dr. Nils Silfverskiold, the noted neurosurgeon wrote Signe on September 29, 1937, with the salutation ''Dear Fellow Student''. He thanked Signe for her visit and for giving the lectures. In reference to Signe's suggestion for an exchange program, Silfverskiold wrote:

> . . . if something like this can be arranged, it would be of interest to us here to have a return visit from your Institute, and for this eventuality, I assure you of my complete cooperation.

In 1938, Signe was officially appointed an Instructor at New York University. Her interest in therapeutic exercise and work at the Hospital for the Ruptured and Crippled helped build her reputation. She was to serve the University until the spring of 1942. Later, in 1948,she joined the faculty of the Institute for Rehabilitation Medicine as a research associate working on a Suction Socket Study sponsored by the Veterans Administration and NYU.

It was in 1938 that Signe was to renew her acquaintance with an individual she had meet many years before. Mary Eleanor Brown, a respected physical therapist, an educator, a writer, and a researcher recalls a personal experience with Signe:

Flash back to the top of the Metropolitan Life Insurance Company in the spacious gymnasium overlooking Madison Square in New York City where I first saw my erstwhile friend and idol Signe. It was a late afternoon in the 1930's and the gym was filling up with employees. I was thrilled to be watching the strong, blonde coach blowing her whistle as a vigorous volley-ball game ensued. These players would be my future clientele I thought, and I even visualized my exercise room off to one side. Always a dancer at heart, I had exhausted Martha Graham with my tormenting insistence on knowing what muscles I needed to call on in order to execute her contorting technic. Then I found not only the Mensendieck System of Functional Exercises, but Bess M. Mensendieck, M.D., its author. Under her eminent self, I started and practiced her system, muscle by muscle, became a teacher, and started a studio of my own. The Metropolitan's enlightened health department was willing to give me a trial, and I was agog to begin right away. Said Signe, "Mensendieck is very fine, but it is a very special system which has been popular in Europe. Americans do not have the discipline. Go to New York University, get your physical education background, come to my muscle-testing classes, see if you like physical therapy. It's a wide open field. It's not restricted in scope. You'll be needed. You will never be out of a job.

Mary Eleanor Brown completed her Master's degree in 1941 at the School of Education, New York University, specializing in posture and body mechanics. It was there that she met Beth Addoms. They became close friends, and it was Mary Eleanor who steered Beth to Dr. George Deaver. It was under his encouragement that Beth Addoms studied physical therapy and became the director of the program at NYU. Mary Eleanor worked for Deaver and taught some classes in the evening. She studied physical therapy at night and on Saturdays and received her certificate in 1945.

Among her classes were those on muscle testing taught by Signe. Deaver also taught in the program, which was attended by physical education and physical therapy students. Signe considered Deaver to be "a good egg" and he, in turn, thought she was the greatest!

Just prior to World War War II, Signe was living very frugally. According to Mary Eleanor Brown:

> She was sympathetic to hard-up students such as myself. She told me she had condensed her belongings, simplified her clothing, ate at the Automats or in her room, and literally lived for work at the hospital. She was, to me, an intellectual giant, the perfect scholar. Her classes and the libraries were home to her. She glowed with every new insight she gained and was an inspiration to all around her.

World War II started in Europe in September, 1939. Signe indicated her routine was "work as usual, NYU, ICD, Dr. Cobb's office, Gould, and Metropolitan Life Insurance night clinic, Dr. Phelp's clinic at A. Harry More School. . . . "

In June 1940, Signe attended the Annual Convention of the American Physiotherapy Association held in Stanford, California, where she participated in a round-table discussion on muscle testing. This discussion led to another article for publication, *Muscle Testing* in the APA Journal (Vol. 21, No.1, 1941).

While Signe worked in the city, she longed to have a quiet place in the country. Her haven was found just outside of Carmel, New York, in Putnam County. On October 4, 1940, she purchased "eight acres of land more or less" from George and Anna Lang off of Bullet Hole Road, in the town of Patterson. A guess as to the total cost, given (in 1986) by the Putnam County Clerk, was $3,500. (This was based on the amount of transfer tax stamps on the deed and their value.) On the site was an old barn and a chicken coop. It was the "coop" that was to be renovated by Signe and made into her first home in the country. The Langs, as neighbors became close friends for more than 30 years. At first, Signe was only able to spend an occasional weekend in Carmel. It took money and time to repair the"coop" and eventually build something more substantial on her land—but it was her land. Over the next 40 years, Signe found refuge on the Bullet Hole Road acreage, enjoying her nature walks, going horseback riding, watching the animals, and working around the area. Finding the most cost-effective construction workers was not easy and it was a common occurrence on a weekend to see Signe on the roof with hammer in hand, or digging a trench or arranging the landscape. It was not until January 16, 1949, that a cinder-block foundation was started for her cottage which was to be her real home. While the coop, the barn and the orchards brought Signe much pleasure, the very site she came to love on Bullet Hole Road would become a major factor many years later in the demise of her physical and mental health.

Another major factor that influenced Signe's choice of escaping to the countryside, was her need for the solitude required for writing. Weekends were spent at the coop, where she communed with nature. Signe's love of nature and animals is depicted in a description of what she saw one night in her yard. Her writing is indicative of the analytical approach she took, her outstanding use of observation and the ability to put it on paper. On two pages torn from a spiral notebook, she wrote:

> February 9, 1941, 10PM . . . Buck long legs and his graceful lady are in the orchard now eating frozen apples and potato peels dumped there by Langs. The moon is nearly full, shinning on the snow and icey slopes. It is almost as light as during the day, but the shadows are blacker and distances seem distorted. The moment I opened the door, I saw four enormously long legs and a dark body . . . or was it a bare spot in the orchard and a couple of branches? Automatically, I leaned backward toward the wall to get my body out of the glaring moonlight and into the shadow of the roof. And there I stood without budging, hardly daring to breathe. Now if thou art a buck, I am going to outstare thee, even though my feet may freeze in the ground while I am waiting. The buck stood like petrified and I knew he was staring at me, although his head was hid-

den in the shadow of the apple tree. But since he heard no more noise and saw no motion, before long he was reassured. He slowly lowered his head to the ground, took a step, scratched the ground, moved again . . . and his whole silhouette stood out sharply against the snow. What a buck! Big like a horse, and what heavy forelegs and shoulders! Like a Moose. Maybe it was a Moose? I didn't think a buck could be that big. Definitely not. Or is it the moonlight that makes him look so fantastic? Now I can hear the snow crack each time he takes a step, but he is in the shadow again. If I move along the wall of the house to the corner, I could see him better. Everything worked out all right and I moved noiseless until—crack—there was some ice breaking under my feet. Instantaneously, the buck caught the noise and off he was over the stone wall. To my surprise, quite close to me, closer than the buck was, there was another deer running away, and I think, a third one further up the hill. That was "graceful lady." She moved much more quietly than Buck Long Legs, and the third one was perhaps a yearling. I decided to take a walk in the moonlight, toward the opposite side so as not to scare the deer family. Ten minutes later when I came back, the Buck was again in the orchard. This time I saw his legs not only like dark branches sticking out of the snow, this time I actually saw the fur on the legs. It was heavy fur and light in color half way down the legs.

In the spring of 1941, on March 25, Signe completed a Red Cross application indicating her interest to do physical therapy in military hospitals. No immediate explanation was given to anyone as to why she decided on such a step. Perhaps she felt the United States would soon be drawn into the world conflict and wanted to take an active role. She may also have seen the opportunity to go "military" which would probably please her father. Nothing happened immediately with her application, so she continued with her work. She prepared a membership report for the American Physiotherapy Association (APA), started a class on body mechanics at NYU, took motion pictures at the Institute for Crippled and Disabled, talked to the P.T. class at New York Hospital about the American Registry for Physical Therapy Technicians, attended a PT conference at the Hotel Pennsylvania, and on April 3, 1941, Signe rented her apartment at 10 East 9th Street and moved to the country house in Carmel.

In the next month, just when planning to go to Walter Reed Hospital in Washington, D.C., to give a lecture, Signe received a radiogram from Ingegerd in Sweden indicating her father, Edvin, had died on May 18. He was buried on May 23 in Helsingborg. Since there was an ocean between Signe and her family, all she could do was fulfill her obligations to her profession. The lecture was given three days later.

Now as a commuter to the city, work continued at N.Y.U. and the Institute for Crippled and Disabled. While at I.C.D. Signe heard of an opening for a physical therapist. She called her friend Mary Eleanor Brown and told her to go see Dr. Deaver at the Institute as he had a 30 dollar-a-month job available! In describing the incident, Mary Eleanor wrote:

> I seized the job, only to loose Signe to the service shortly thereafter. I wanted to join the Navy. When Dr. Deaver heard about that, he told me ''NO.'' You are drafted for work here at ICD, to help with the courses for enlisted men of the armed forces of the United States and Canada who will man the rehabilitation centers for the wounded soldiers. You are Signe Brunnstrom's replacement. A laughable assignment for one who wasn't then even a physical therapist!

The United States went to war on December 7, 1941. The new year was to bring about a major change in Signe Brunnstrom's life. The Red Cross took action on her application, and she responded to the call to duty to serve her newly-adopted country.

Chapter Three

The War Years

The call to duty came through the Red Cross. A "discontinuance slip" at Metropolitan Life Insurance, dated August 28, 1942, states, "volunteered for duty in the American Red Cross. To be stationed at Sheppard Field, Texas."

Signe, as a civilian physical therapist was assigned to the the Station Hospital, Army Air Corps, Sheppard Field, Wichita Falls, Texas—quite a change from the excitement of New York City. Apparently, she accepted the assignment with great anticipation and expectations of an unusual experience. It was to be a year of many activities, some travel, meeting new friends and learning how the military service functions. Signe described her August 30 trip to Texas and duty at Sheppard Field in a spiral composition notebook which was maintained as her diary:

> Grand style travelling, all seats in the plane taken, mostly Army officers. Overnight trip to Ft. Worth, arrived 9:05 AM, seemed no distance at all. Beautiful moonlight night. In the morning, above the clouds, sunshine. At all landings, curtains were drawn, we arrived "blindfolded" at every airport. War time regulations. Local bus Fort Worth to Wichita Falls packed. Rangers in big hats and magnificent leather belts kept

> piling in and it got hotter and hotter. Under the glaring Texas sun the bus kept rolling on, miles and miles, and more miles over straight mountainous roads. It seemed as if we were going to the end of the world.

Despite the heat and lack of comfort, Signe saw beauty in her surroundings. She wrote:

> The country is pretty flat, few cultivated fields and far between the ranges. Dry looking pastures, scattered oaks and willow trees, white and purple cactus bushes, horses, mules, cows. Bright brick colored dust roads taking off at right angles from the main road. A swamp and two bright white herons . . .

Arriving in Wichita Falls, Signe obtained a room at the biggest hotel, The Kemp. Her description of it reads, "dreary, only moderately clean place, rooms ranged from $2.25 to $3.75, badly kept, old worn out furniture." She decided to find an apartment, but after hours of walking, it was the same result everywhere: " . . . Sorry, it's just been rented earlier today." Wichita Falls was overflowing with soldiers!

Sheppard Field was about five miles from town. It took 30 minutes by bus. Signe was to report on September 1 at 8am to building 1210 of the Station Hospital. The Army Air Forces Technical Command was housed at Sheppard Field. According to Signe, "an estimated 65,000 enlisted men and officers turned the field into a little town in itself." She described how her time was allocated on the first day: "filling out forms, endless papers, getting a physical examination, fingerprinting, photograph taken, getting official pass to the field, etc."

On her way back to the hotel, Signe decided she would get a car:

> I stopped at a second hand car place in the afternoon. I saw a 1939 Plymouth for $495. The salesman and owner of the place proposed a date for tonight—wanted to show me the country around Wichita Falls.

Fast work! Most people are very friendly, some a little too friendly it seems.

Before I recount Signe's arrival in the Physical Therapy Department at Sheppard, there is a story to be told by another physical therapist, Mary G. Flickinger, of Hinsdale, Illinois:

In March 1942, I signed up as a physical therapist to serve in the U.S. Army. I was assigned to the Station Hospital in Sheppard Field, Texas. This was at a time when the only women in the services were nurses. Physical therapists were civilian employees. (However, a bill eventually was passed commissioning therapists and it went into effect a year later).

I had just received my certificate in physical therapy from Northwestern University in February 1942 and the Army was my first job. I arrived at Sheppard Field to discover the physical therapy department consisted of one whole ward of the station hospital. There were seven treatment tables, one Hubbard tank, one leg and arm whirlpool, six heat lamps and an ultraviolet lamp. That was the extent of my equipment. Six enlisted men were assigned to physical therapy and the only treatment they administered was to turn a heat lamp on a patient for twenty minutes. There was no physical therapist so no one received exercises. About eighty patients a day were going through the department. Most of them were victims of the obstacle course and many had post-operative knee conditions. There I was, green out of school, with no experience and having to cope with a situation like that. However, I did get a program set up. I trained several of the medics to give a simple massage and to administer routine exercises. I personally treated the complicated injuries. Had I been older and more experienced, I probably would have been defeated by the enormity of the job and I couldn't have gotten the job done. I went to the Commander of the hospital and requested a desperately needed assistant. After several months of waiting, I was notified that my new assistant was to arrive sometime in the summer. Can you imagine my delight—but also my embarrassment—when the new assistant turned out to be SIGNE BRUNNSTROM? There I was, the "rookie", straight out of school with Signe.

On September 2, Mary Flickinger was ill and in the hospital. It was necessary for Signe to take over. Signe recalled the situation:

> I had to jump in right away. My job is to boss around six privates in the medical corps. All have a short hospital training and have learned a little about massage and heat. They are all awfully nice boys and they expect to do all the work. One is in hydro, one making arch supports, one in the office, and the other three do heat, ultra violet and massage. A large number of patients are diagnosed low back strain, myositis, arthritis,—too complicated cases wouldn't do for the Army.

Signe's ability to analyze a problem found one soldier whose diagnosis was "myositis" actually had a "typical scalenus anterior syndrome with cervical rib." One of the first things she decided to do was to talk to the physician in charge. He was an orthopedist, Dr. Cole, who had visited the department once since April 1. Signe tried to talk with him but according to Signe "he was too busy, told me just to go ahead." So that's what she decided to do.

Mary Flickinger and Signe worked together the rest of the year and were very close to one another and to the medic enlisted men. Mary wrote:

> We were a little family, Signe, myself, the dental hygienist, and our six enlisted men. All of us were away from family and friends so we clung together. Since we weren't in the Army at that time, we were allowed to live off of post. Signe bought an old beat-up car and she hauled us about. Gasoline was rationed so we begged and borrowed coupons whenever possible so we could use the car and that was great fun. At least once

a week we went horse back riding. Off we went galloping through the mesquite and the Texas bush. Signe was an accomplished rider and knew how to ride formation so she whipped us all into shape to do some formation riding. We also went on picnics, had outdoor BBQ's and Swedish pancake suppers at Signe's. All of these activities were a great diversion from the humdrum day-in and day-out life where one was isolated on an Army post.

Signe also lined us up every noon so that we could do calisthenics. Following that exercise, we had anatomy review with Signe teaching us. Imagine the poor medics trying to absorb all of that with their limited backgrounds. One had been a cowboy, one a cook, a butcher, a truck driver, a stock-boy, and fortunately one an O.T. These types of activities underlined Signe's constant and on-going search for knowledge and the application of her own drive for furthering her views on education. There was no one making any of us do these things and I have carried with me in my professional career her inspiration for constant improvement.

At the end of our year's duty as civilian PT's, we could no longer stay in the Army, unless we enlisted. I left to join my husband in Enid, Oklahoma, where he was stationed. I only saw Signe once through these intervening years when she lectured in Chicago many years ago, but I shall never forget her as an exceptional person as well as a true professional.

On Sunday, September 6, Signe wandered around town taking a look at the Post Office, the Public Library (it was closed until 3 pm), and getting acquainted with the USO. She was impressed with the USO's work in organizing meetings, dances and concerts. It was at the USO's facility that she met Alfred Zigler. Signe described the meeting:

I had a long chat with a fellow from Oregon who told me practically his whole life story and that of his family. Having traveled all around the world for a firm delivering technical equipment to the government, in-

> stalling it in all corners of the world, he finally got a job in the home office, settled down with his family in a home of his own, only to be drafted in April. Now, he is a private at the technical school. Tomorrow, Labor Day, he is going to show me around the post, the school buildings being open to the public. He also invited me to join the Java Club which meets every Sunday 9 am to eat doughnuts and drink coffee. Private Zigler (Dutch descent) is well educated, well read, writes short stories and poems. One of his poems appeared in the USO's paper.

The next day, Signe made a short stop in the P.T. department and then went around the field with Private Zigler. He showed her a typical barracks where she found ''everything tip-top—in perfect order for inspection.'' Later they went to several hangars where Signe was impressed with the amount of equipment made available for the education of the personnel. A visit to the Service Club followed. There she met Al's friends, including one who in private life was a sculptor. The service club's restaurant was crowded so Al and Signe took a bus to town and had a nice dinner, '' . . . Al talking and talking as if he hadn't had a chance to talk to anybody for weeks.'' Afterwards, they saw a movie—''Sergeant York'' with Gary Cooper. ''It was almost 6 pm before I said good-bye to Al and we certainly had spent a nice day together.''

A week later, Signe spent another day with Al. First at the ''Java Club'', and later, at 1 pm, they went out to dinner. ''It was swell,'' Signe wrote, ''listening to Al telling me how he organized the lumber industry in Oregon or was it Alaska?'' They hiked around the residential section of town, went to the USO, played ping-pong and attended a vesper service. Then it was ''out with Al and Roy Geoghegan for a drink.'' Despite the problems with living quarters, transportation, the Texas heat and military service, Signe apparently, for a short time, found someone to whom she could relate. Unfortunately the relationship did not last long, as her diary indicates her close friend had been shipped out: ''November 6, Al Zigler in Santa Monica, California.''

Signe adapted to the military post gradually. Whatever she encountered, she noted in her diary as a new learning experience:

> I am getting used to the terms and expressions. "P.X." is Post Exchange where one can buy sodas and other drinks, cigarettes, writing paper, etc. "K.P." is kitchen police, in other words, kitchen duty. "Gold-bricks" are patients who don't want to get well, they would rather come to their physiotherapy than to drilling. And they do escape calisthenics which apparently is torture to many. It seems as if it really were a torture considering all the sprained backs which result from it.
>
> I also learned how to handle a cafeteria tray in the mess hall. We do get ordinary plates, cups and glasses and not a mess kit. "You may take all the food you want, but eat all you take" says the poster at the counter. However, in true American fashion, huge quantities are left on the plates and thrown out.

Signe seemed to enjoy the surroundings and saw great beauty in the landscape, not only in natural items but also in man-made structures. She described the landscape as follows:

> It is very beautiful in the morning when going out to the Post. After leaving town, we pass the CONOCO refineries on the right hand side. What a sight! Dozens of black bordered shining silver gray tanks spread across a huge area. Their enormous silver balls, chimneys, pipe lines and what not, all illuminated by the rising sun. On the left hand side, the panhandle oil-wells and refineries in gray and red offer a similar view though less brilliant. Further out on the plains the silhouettes of more wells are seen far away. I begin to love the plains in the early morning before the sun has risen high. The sky and the plains offer delicate shades of blue, green, brown and there is a peculiar serenity. There is nothing to obstruct your view and your eyes can take it all in . . . the wide horizon, the quietness,

> and serenity of the plains, the cleanliness of the air as the last darkness of the night disappears. You can even look at the rising sun without hurting your eyes, the same sun that a few hours later has transformed the landscape into an unbearably hot, dry, glaring stretch of land, which you cannot look at unless you wear dark glasses.

On another occasion, in October, Signe went horseback riding on "ranch 77." Again she approached the sights most poetically:

> I began to see the beauty of the prairie. When the sun is setting or early in the morning, the prairie is wonderful; delicate colors, flowers, insects, birds the like of which I have never seen before. Hello, you funny Jack rabbit with your big donkey ears and long legs. Aren't you afraid of a rider? No, he hops away wiggling his enormous ears. The saddle is creaking in a comforting way, old "Shaw" who is a "gaited" horse is quite willing and very sure-footed. Western saddle, blue-jeans as riding outfit, real cowboy style. What are those enormous hawks with a white stripe across the tail? Gee, they certainly are circling low by now, can see their eagle eyes and powerful beaks.

In the physical therapy department, patients came and went. Some special cases were noted by Signe in her diary, such as William Mansfield Jennings. He was post-op reconstruction of the knee. Signe noted:

> . . . leg in bad shape, quadriceps-hip flexor paralysis. After a few weeks treatment, one gets to know the patients very well. What wouldn't I give to see his cattle ranch in Utah. . . . 62,000 acres, 100 horses, 2,000 head of cattle, 6,000 sheep. That's the kind of thing one sees in the movies. "Utah" is a college graduate, has played on football team, has 1,400 hours of flying. Loves his ranch, is a real cowboy at heart. A fine boy. I am working hard with him but no improvement of the paralyzed muscles.

(In an attempt to locate Jennings in 1986, I wrote the Veterans Affairs Department in Salt Lake City. There being no such department in the capital, my letter was referred to the Veterans Benefit Coordinator of Social Services. Thanks to the efforts of Delores Busch, Coordinator, I was told Jennings died on June 9, 1978 and is buried in Sunset Gardens, Draper, Utah.)

Additional comments about patients demonstrated the close attachment Signe developed with many of the servicemen:

> Leahy (with the mysterious tibialis palsy) is off for Officers Training School. Traynor (dislocated 5th finger) still waiting on Officer Candidate School. Colonel Clagget, Commanding Officer of the field, comes for treatment every other day. All time high in physio, 123 patients. Finally had a talk with Lt. Lambert, orthopedic surgeon. He doesn't think much about physio—will come around sooner or later, I hope.

Another physical therapist who served in the Army and knew Signe was Major Mary J. Torp of Del City, Oklahoma. She recalled that while at Sheppard Field, Signe was called the "Sergeant P.T.", and her twenty-five-year-old boss "the Corporal P.T.". According to Major Torp, Signe was interested in accepting a commission in the Army after completing her role with the Red Cross. Signe planned to meet with Major Emma Vogel in Washington, D.C. on the way home to New York at the end of March, (1943).

On April 1, Signe left Sheppard Field and traveled via Dallas to Memphis. She described part of this experience in her diary:

> Because of floods, missed my train to Atlanta. I was going to visit Warm Springs Foundation. Stayed all day in Memphis, watching the riverboats on the Mississippi, walked through the colored section. Night train to Washington,D.C., soldiers, sailors and marines jammed the train, sleeping in corridors on their bags and on top of each other. No Pullman could be had, so

I sat on my gluteus maximus for a whole night and whole day, until that part of my anatomy was as worn out as had been my feet the day before. The waiting line in the dining car was as bad as the line-up for the orthopedic clinic on a Wednesday at Sheppard Field!

Arriving at Union Station in Washington, D.C., Signe was overwhelmed with the rush of people. She said it was "like the New York subways during rush hours." She took a cab to the Office of the Surgeon General to keep a scheduled meeting with Major Vogel. Signe described her as "a terrifically important looking brass-beladen, blue uniformed lady major." It must have been quite a meeting!

Signe described the session honestly and with keen perception:

> I got an ice-cold reception and was told that there was no chance for me serving with the Army since I had just passed the age limit (Signe was 45). Nothing she or anybody else could do about it. Previous service on an Army Post does not count since military status of P.T.'s just went into effect.

Years later Signe told Mary Torp that she was anxious to accept a commission in the Army until she met Major Vogel in Washington. With the reception she received and the attitude displayed by Major Vogel, Signe obviously was turned off to the Army. However, she had another plan through which she could serve in the military. At the recruiting station of the WAVES, news was better. Signe wrote:

> My application filed in Dallas had been approved. I was to report for training with a May 10th group and there is a job waiting for me at the conclusion of the O.T.S. So it looks as if my Army days were over . . . now the NAVY!

The next two months were spent at home at the Bullet Hole. The weather was very cold and there was a snowstorm in April. Signe made the decision to join the Navy and was able to arrange for someone to take over her home while away.

On June 5, she reported to Northampton, Massachusetts and Mt. Holyoke College for indoctrination at the U.S. Naval Midshipmen's Training School. She graduated from the program on July 27, 1943, and received a commission as a Lieutenant Junior Grade. Her orders were to report to the Naval Hospital at Mare Island, California by August 5.

When Lt. Brunnstrom arrived at Mare Island, she found a functioning department of physical therapy under the direction of First Class Pharmacist Mate Robert A. Teckemeyer. (In his professional physical therapy career, Teckemeyer was to become the Associate Executive Director of Administration, for the American Physical Therapy Association in Alexandria, Virginia.) Recalling those days in World War II, Teckemeyer wrote on February 20,1985:

> I enlisted in the Navy in 1942 following graduation from the University of Wisconsin and certification as a physical therapist. Susanne Hirt was one of my classmates. After six months practicing as a PT at Wisconsin General Hospital, I enlisted at Great Lakes Naval Station and soon found myself with orders to Mare Island Hospital at Vallejo, California. I was named director of the physical therapy department. When Signe arrived as a Lt. J.G. she was assigned director of the department. Between the two of us we established a Navy P.T. school for some twenty corpsmen to teach some basic science and PT techniques as well as treatment of all cases sent to the department.

Lucy Gore Stead, now living in Vancouver, British Columbia, was an occupational therapist with the Navy. She recalled her service days:

> When I first arrived at Mare Island in June 1943, Signe was functioning in very inadequate space, under a Lt. Commander Doctor of Physical Medicine and with two assistants. I was next door, also with two assistants and for the next several months we stumbled a bit, doing straight orthopedic work and figuring how to work effectively and I, with not too much experi-

ence, started to learn from Signe. She was my mentor and friend during the years from 1943–1946. It was a period of both personal and professional growth for all of us, and the friendships we made were strong and lasting ones. Shirley Mainwaring (an x-ray technician) and I knew Signe best. Signe and Jean Campbell (an educational services officer, ex-English teacher and librarian) had the only two cars. They saved up precious gas and five or six of us had two weekend junkets to Yosemite and to Lake Tahoe. Natalie Kahn was the psychologist and has remained my closest friend. There was also Mabel Powers, an education officer. We were a close and friendly group of W.A.V.E. officers.

A major change was to take place at Mare Island in which Signe would be a most prominent figure. In October 1943, a physician, Henry H. Kessler, Captain, USN, arrived to initiate a new plan that would make Mare Island the West Coast center for amputees. Until that time, according to Teckemeyer, "the department caseload was the usual war injuries, orthopedic, neurological, burns plus a number of polio patients."

Kessler, in his 1968 autobiography, *The Knife is Not Enough*, described the changes he brought about and the new program:

> Although I had been transferred to Mare Island as an orthopedic surgeon, I was vitally concerned with the development of a complete program of rehabilitation services: vocational guidance, counseling and training, and education for a return to civilian life. I spoke to Captain Owen (the Commanding Officer) about this, and he agreed. We created a small organization with Lieutenant Henry Lindgren as educational officer, Miss Signe Brunnstrom as physical therapy officer, Miss Lucy Gore as occupational therapy officer, Miss Natalie Kahn as psychologist, and two volunteers, Mrs. Evelyn Garden and W. A. Huggins.

Dr. Kessler used all kinds of innovative methods to make the amputee center a success. He raised funds, did public relations, spoke at various groups, sought employment for the amputees and personally became involved with many of the wounded men. He was the driving force in establishing the center. Lucy Gore Stead speaks of the many changes that came about when Dr. Kessler took over:

> When he arrived upon the scene as Chief of Orthopedics and Rehabilitation, things began to take off. A new building went up, we got better space and our staff mushroomed, still mostly untrained hospital corpsmen (though selected carefully) who had to be taught what to do. Signe was a marvelous teacher and undaunted. By now the casualties from the Pacific Island landings were rolling in and I have always felt it was one of my luckiest strikes having Signe by my side in this somewhat scary assignment for a fairly inexperienced O.T. We were fortunate in having Henry Kessler too. He knew how to push us and be supportive at the same time, and wove a a tightly knit and closely cooperating rehabilitation department. The doctor of physical medicine left and Signe and I were put directly under Dr. Kessler. He chaired weekly rehab meetings of heads of all the relevant departments. We discussed cases and plotted strategy. A prosthetics shop was set up and we began treating men and teaching them to use their prostheses. Before long we discovered that too many men were going home on leave with their appliances in their suitcases instead of on their bodies, especially the arm amputees. We weren't about to accept this as inevitable after all our hard work, so it was mutually decided to invoke naval discipline. We developed an achievement test, printed it in the O.T. shop, and discharge was withheld until each man could pass it. I was given the unenviable job of enforcing this and making ourselves even more unpopular. At Signe's instigation penalties were introduced for missed physiotherapy appointments. There was a certain amount of amusement over the sight of a five-foot WAVE (me) hauling great strapping Marines before the Captain to be called down for missing P.T. The men grumbled but in the end, more or

> less, they accepted the sense of it and really put up with us very well. I do remember one party that Signe gave for staff and some patients, where I was taxed by one sailor, plaintively and half-seriously, on the wrong-headedness of WAVE officers as slave drivers instead of being 'Angels of Mercy.' Those who knew Signe will recognize her influence in this no-nonsense approach. They were good years for all of us, with a sense of shared purpose, a feeling of doing an important job and a lot of learning in the process. Signe, in her unpretentious way, was a key part of all of this, for me at least. She really developed the principles of aftercare for amputees at Mare Island, and taught us all. She worked very hard and was an amazing combination of driving intensity and cheerful vitality.

In between all of the work, Signe did find some time to go horseback riding and hiking. She also enjoyed a good party. She notes this in her diary following a meeting of the American Physiotherapy Association in San Francisco (May 4,1944). Dr. Kessler participated in the program and spoke on amputations. After the meeting, they went to the apartment of one of the officers where, according to Signe, "plenty of drinks were served." On another occasion, she recalls attending a "fiesta" at Father Burne's church, "dancing, gambling, beer drinking." Bob Teckemeyer also had many opportunities to socialize with Signe. He and his wife Fran had a small apartment directly above Signe's apartment, on the beach and near the Naval base. While regulations precluded fraternization between officers and other personnel, Signe, Bob and Fran spent many evenings at one or another's apartment over cocktails and dinner, talking shop and discussing the department's patient load. Bob remembers that Signe "enjoyed people and a good time and specifically parties." Describing some of the social activities, he wrote:

> She was a good sport and athletically inclined. She did smoke and really enjoyed a good cigar after dinner. Signe loved hearing and telling a good joke and was an

> excellent story teller. Due to her Swedish heritage she created an international flavor to all that she came in contact with and was well liked by everyone.

Summarizing his personal relationship with Signe, Bob stated:

> She was an excellent teacher and demanded perfection from herself and those around her. I can attribute a great deal of my success in the profession to the knowledge I gained from Signe both from our professional and social contact. My contact with her following the war was only a card and a note at Christmas and the occasional professional visit to the west coast APTA meetings. When in the San Francisco bay area she would either call or be my guest in my home in Santa Rosa.

The psychologist in the department, Natalie Kahn, is now Natalie Zucker of Santa Fe Springs, California. In a June 1985 letter, she wrote:

> I was the psychologist in that happy band of WAVE officers at Mare Island. Although we were professionals, Signe was the essence of professionalism and a model for the younger of us to emulate. I can see her in my mind's eye hurrying down the hospital corridor, body bent forward like a skier going downhill. She had so much to accomplish in her lifetime. She was strong, sinewy, and the epitome of integrity. I viewed her as a strong oak tree. I was not close to Signe. We shared the common experiences of working together, but the age difference put us in different generations. Also, she was a private person and I had the sense that she did not encourage closeness . . . I honor her memory.

Alice Berg, P.T., of Waukesha, Wisconsin, also was at Mare Island in 1945–46. On September 17, 1984 she wrote:

> Signe was an inspiration to all of us. She was ever the teacher with a most inquiring mind. I remember

one day, she was demonstrating muscle action to a doctor using a person rather than a drawing or other aid. The doctor very enthusiastically said, "THIS IS LIVING ANATOMY!" He was very impressed as we all were.

As an extra duty assignment, Signe accepted the responsibility to accompany some staff with 15 male and four female patients to Washington, D.C. The date was May 5, 1944. In four days, the group arrived without incident at Bethesda Naval Hospital. Signe reported to the Bureau of Medicine and Surgery rushed to the Bureau of Personnel in Arlington and returned to Bethesda. She then had some leave time and just made a night train to New York. May 10 and the following weekend Signe spent relaxing at her "Bullet Hole" country home. She kept busy every minute as indicated in the following:

> Fruit trees in bloom, bulbs out, Lillies of the Valley and lilacs beginning. Spoke to the Langs about their woodland property. Went over my property checking on blueprints. Last day transplanted a maple to the west side of the barn.

Once again she arranged for someone to spend the summer of 1944 at her small home. Then it was back to New York City to attend the APTA conference at the Hotel Pennsylvania, May 19–21. On the twenty second, she reported again to the Bureau of Medicine and boarded a train for the west coast. By Friday the 26th, Signe was back at work on Mare Island.

In between her travels, treating patients and teaching staff, Signe found time to give some lectures in the professional community. She described one particular trip:

> 8 August 1944 . . . Lucy Gore, Jean Campbell and myself to Stanford University to speak on rehabilitation. Were met by Hazel Furscott in San Francisco who drove us to Palo Alto. Lectured two hours to P.T. class. Among those present were Catherine Worthingham,

Lucille Daniels and Lt. Kennedy, former patient at Mare Island. Dinner at Catherine's.

In a letter of January 25, 1985, commenting on the preparation of Signe's biography, Lucille Daniels wrote:

> We (Catherine Worthingham and I) had great respect for her clinical competence at Morrison Rehabilitation Center and for her activities as teacher and author. Her fine contributions to the profession of physical therapy earned the respect of related members of the academic community such as anatomists as well as orthopedists and surgeons.

Back in New York in September, 1944, Althea M. Jones (formerly an Associate Professor, of Physical Therapy at Columbia University,) entered the Hospital for Special Surgery to study physical therapy. Signe was supposed to teach the course but since she was in the Navy, a substitute teacher was engaged. Althea recalled those days in a letter of February 5, 1986:

> We as students were asked to read Signe's article on the action of the gastrocnemius on the ankle and the knee. Her careful analysis of the muscle action was exciting to read and I remember the enlightening discussion the article precipitated. Her writing made a profound impression on me and throughout my career has been a major influence on my thought.

Although busy with her various assignments, Signe maintained her diary and noted the important events of the time, in far away places, such as the liberation of Paris, the capture of Marseilles, peace in Rumania and sinking of the U.S.S. Birmingham. She also was very concerned with recording the impact of casualties at Mare Island:

> 23 August: Amputees keep coming in from Saipan. Now Ward 14, 15, 19, A, B, C are filled to the last bunk. Bombing of the Philippines continues. 16 October: Ward 21 and 26 have been added to the orthopedic service. Patients are flown in from the islands via Pearl

> Harbor and Hamilton Field and reach Mare Island in less than forty-eight hours. Guam casualties have been heavy. Pelu injured now coming in.

Signe's work was recognized as being exceptional. On the first day of November, 1944, she was promoted to the rank of Lieutenant in the Medical Service Corps, Naval Reserve of the U.S. The appointment certificate was signed by Francis P. Matthews, Secretary of the Navy. To celebrate the promotion, Captain and Mrs. Greer hosted a party for Signe at the Officers' Club. Among those present were Captain Kessler, Dr. D.T. Toffelmier, Dr. Paul Olson, Lt. Jessie Phillips, Lt. Lucy Gore and Lt. Natalie Kahn.

In the midst of all of the work, Signe managed to find time to write an article and become involved in the preparation of some films. The article, *Physical Therapy in the Aftercare of Amputations of the Lower Extremity* appeared in the U.S. Naval Medical Bulletin, (43: 634–644, 1944). A copy was sent by Signe's New York friend, physical therapist Margit Aden, on November 22 to the APTA Executive Secretary, Mildred Elson. Margit also informed APTA that Signe had been promoted. Mildred Elson wrote Signe on November 27:

> Miss Aden was kind enough to send me a copy of your article. It was really excellent, and we are all terribly proud of you and your progress. You are our one bright spot in the Navy. I do hope we may reprint this or have an original article from you. With very good wishes for your continued advancement.

Signe had further correspondence with Mildred Elson in which she expressed her concern for physical therapy not being represented in the Navy's Bureau of Medicine and Surgery. She wrote Miss Elson at the national office at 1790 Broadway, New York City, on January 24, 1945:

> I wonder if you know that the Occupational Therapists have managed to place a member of their association as a consultant at the Bureau of Medicine and Surgery Navy Department, Washington, D.C.? She

was an Ensign, when appointed and has recently been promoted to full Lieutenant. We too need a representative desperately, and unless and until we get one, we will not be able to go far. There is too much red tape for anything that comes from me to reach the persons in Washington they are intended to reach. I have made reports every time I get a chance to, but all my efforts have been in vain.

I wish we could get someone like Hazel Furscott to represent Physical Therapy at the Bureau. I am convinced that she is the right person. Do you think our association could do something about this matter?

As you undoubtedly know, the Navy needs qualified physiotherapists very badly. Yet, the Procurement Office in San Francisco, apparently in accordance with orders from the above, turns down every applicant. I know personally of two members of our association who have been turned down twice. They would need a waiver for their eyes, and it shouldn't be impossible to get, but the office refused even to try.

The training of P.T. assistants in the Navy is another sore spot, and it has given me plenty of trouble. Everything in connection with P.T. in the Navy is very unsatisfactory. What can we do about it? The fact that P.T. is very much appreciated by our Chief of Surgery and Chief of Orthopedics helps me personally, but it doesn't solve our problems.

A note on the letter indicates Miss Elson referred the matter to the APTA's Advisory Committee.

The two films photographed by Navy communications personnel were completed by 1945. One was entitled "Aftercare of Leg Amputations," (16mm, silent, color, running time about one hour.) The other was "Peripheral Nerve Injuries," (16 mm, silent, color, approximately 20 minutes.) The premiere showing of "Aftercare of Leg Amputations" was held February 2, 1945 before a general staff meeting. Captain Owen and the medical and surgical staff were present. Guests included Mrs. Nimitz, Mrs. Tisdale and Mrs.

Owen. Signe served as the narrator. Two weeks later, Signe and Lucy Gore, O.T., attended an APTA meeting in San Francisco. Signe presented her film and Lucy showed "Aftercare of Upper Extremity Amputations." Both were very well received. Signe's film was used for some time after the war, but unfortunately it was lost in the mail.

In spite of Signe's feeling that there were many unsatisfactory situations in the Navy, she continued to give her effort to improving the treatment protocol for amputees, training the personnel, lecturing in the professional community, serving on committees and writing. She also noted more important events in her diary, such as:

> 19 Feb. Marines hit the beach at Iwo Jima. 12 April, President Roosevelt dies at Warm Springs,Ga. 25 April, World Security Conference held in San Francisco. 26 April, Russians in Berlin.

The war was nearing a conclusion.

Jack Hofkosh, of New York, met Signe for the first time while serving as a Naval Hospital Corpsman in 1945. "I had been assigned for six weeks as an Amputee Rehabilitation Specialist at Oak Knoll Naval Hospital, Oakland, California. The WAVE Lieutenant responsible for the program was Signe Brunnstrom," Jack wrote in a letter of August 11, 1987. After leaving California he developed and headed an amputee rehabilitation program at the Naval Hospital in Philadelphia. "Meeting Signe and the assignment in Philadelphia were the most important factors for my pursuing training as a physical therapist upon discharge from the Navy in 1947." In 1950, Jack Hofkosh graduated from New York University, worked at the N.Y.U. Institute for Rehabilitation Medicine and served as the Director of Physical Therapy in the facility for 33 years. Signe and Jack were destined to work together again at the Institute in 1956.

After three years of service to the Navy, Signe was about to receive appropriate recognition. On November 14, 1945, Captain C. W. Ross, Medical Officer-in-Charge of the Naval Hospital at Mare Island, wrote a memo to the Navy Bureau of Personnel in Washington. The subject was Lt. Signe Brunnstrom and the Award of the Medal of Merit. He wrote:

> 1. Since reporting for duty at this hospital on 5 August 1943, subject officer has been in charge of the physical therapy department of this hospital. This department has functioned as a rehabilitation activity since April 1944.
>
> 2. Lieutenant Brunnstrom through her professional skill has inspired the entire staff of the rehabilitation program by her steadfast and selfless devotion to duty. Her enthusiasm for her work has stimulated patients to put forth increasingly greater efforts in accelerating their own physical rehabilitation.
>
> 3. In view of the foregoing it is considered that Lieutenant Brunnstrom has performed meritorious service both as a trained physical therapist and as an instructor in physical therapy, thereby contributing by her own outstanding performance of duty incalculable benefit to the Navy and the United States in the rehabilitation of amputees and other war casualty patients, which is considered to have been performed in an outstanding manner well beyond the high standard normally to be expected.

It would be some time before the Navy took action on commending Signe for her work.

For New Year's 1946, Signe visited Seattle, and returned to Mare Island on January 4. Throughout the winter and through the spring she maintained her busy schedule, which included meeting with representatives of the Committee on Prosthetic Devices, starting a library project for the committee at the University of California Medical School, consulting in the gait clinic at the Naval Hospital, showing her motion picture, organizing a filing system for literature review, reorganizing the rehabilitation program, completing the job analysis for Navy therapists and holding barracks duty. She also managed some time to carry out research and prepare two articles for submission to the Physiotherapy Review. One was: *Comparative Strength of Muscles with Simi-*

lar Function, a study of Peripheral Nerve Injuries of the Upper Extremity. It was published in 1946, (Vol.26 No. 2). The other article, *Walking Training of the Amputee: Some Biomechanical Considerations,* was published in the Physiotherapy Review (Vol. 27, No. 3) in 1947.

Two disappointments were noted in her diary. The first involved some travel. She was invited to attend a meeting in Chicago on prosthetic devices but could not get the military orders to go. The second, was on a cultural note. A concert to be given at the hospital by the world-famous pianist, Jose Iturbi, was canceled!

Socially, there was a farewell party on February 3 for Bob and Fran Teckemeyer. The Navy lost one of its most effective physical therapy personnel.

On April 2, 1946, Signe received notice of her release from active duty. A letter from Captain Ross of the hospital stated:

> On the occasion of your release from active duty I desire to express my appreciation of the services which you have rendered to the Navy in time of war. During your assignment as Physiotherapist from 4 Aug. 1943, to 2 April 1946, you performed your duties in a manner which met the high standards of the Naval Service. The officer like qualities and professional ability which you displayed have contributed materially to the successful performance of the mission of this command.
>
> It is my hope that you will meet every success on your return to civilian life.

While Signe may have been very pleased, it was apparent that it was a form letter with her name and dates placed in the appropriate blank spaces—typical of the military!

The important letter, dated April 4, 1946, came from the Secretary of the Navy, James Forrestal. It was a commendation letter and citation:

> The Secretary of the Navy takes pleasure in commending
>
> Lieutenant Signe Brunnstrom

United States Naval Reserve

for service as set forth in the following CITATION:

For outstanding service as Officer-in-Charge of the Physical Therapy Department, United States Naval Hospital, Mare Island, California, from August 1943 to October 1945. Acting as a trained physical therapist and as an instructor in physical therapy. Lieutenant Brunnstrom, by her enthusiasm, stimulated patients to put forth increasingly greater efforts in accelerating their physical rehabilitation. Her skill, sympathetic understanding and determination were of incalculable benefit in the rehabilitation of amputees and other war casualties and her steadfast performance of duty reflects the highest credit upon Lieutenant Brunnstrom and the United States Naval Service. A copy of this citation has been made a part of Lieutenant Brunnstrom's official record, and she is hereby authorized to wear the Commendation ribbon.

Evidently someone paid attention to the memo Captain Ross sent to the Bureau of Personnel in November 1945. One could imagine how proud Signe's father, Colonel Brunnstrom would have been to know his daughter received such a military commendation.

While still in the service, Signe attended the APTA conference in Monterey. A new physical therapist at the conference that day was Susanne Hirt, who later made major outstanding contributions to the education of physical therapists and now is the Physical Therapy Professor Emeritus at the Medical College of Virginia-Virginia Commonwealth University.

Signe was my first outstanding role model. I met her the first time at our National Conference in California in 1946. It was my very first conference and Signe was still in the Navy. She appeared on stage in her white Navy uniform and gave a very unusual professional presentation of her work with amputees during the war. At that moment, I remember I felt I was in the right profession. Even though I never worked with Signe on a

> continued close basis, we met a number of times at workshops and somehow, managed to develop a quite intimate feeling towards each other. It may be that our foreign accents and some other slight similarities in background helped create this.

The three years in the service proved to be very profitable for the indomitable Signe. She gained stature as a therapist, a rehabilitation specialist, a leader, a teacher, an author, a lecturer, a researcher and an activist in the profession of physical therapy. Though she didn't know it in 1946, much of Signe's successful work and approach to the treatment of amputees would be the basis for her first book.

In addition, her contact with Dr.. Henry Kessler would lead to one of her major gainful work experiences in 1949. Overall, the discipline and the command seen in the Naval service influenced Signe in many aspects of her work. She enjoyed the Navy and the role she played in giving service to her adopted country. On April 3, 1946, Lt. Signe Brunnstrom reported to Balboa Park (California) for separation from the Navy.

Chapter Four

The Fulbright Scholar

The return trip to New York started on April 20, 1946. Signe's first stop was in Ogden, Utah, where she visited the Physical Therapy Department at Bushnell General Hospital. She then spent some time in Chicago and Evanston and finally arrived at Bullet Hole Road on May 5. There was a lot of work to be done around the house and on the land. For a short period, Signe devoted her time to becoming reacquainted with the countryside. About two weeks later, she was back on the lecture circuit with a talk and presentation of the amputee film at the APTA's New York chapter. Just after that, Signe's personal record of activities states, "no more entries . . . believe I went to Sweden."

The payroll records of Metropolitan Life Insurance confirm Signe's next big activity. An entry, signed by "Ray" on October 30, 1946 states:

> Miss Brunnstrom saw me today after returning from a trip to Sweden. She said that because she could not be assigned a satisfactory position at New York University she had decided to locate in San Francisco, so that she was no longer interested in returning to us.

In a letter of December 16, 1946, to Barbara White, Executive Secretary of the APTA, Signe wrote:

> My trip west was delayed for a long time, but I am finally leaving on December 18. I am stopping over at Cleveland and Chicago and then will go on to San Francisco.

In the same letter, Signe showed her pride in her little home on Bullet Hole Road when she wrote:

> I now have a bathroom in the "coop", but it took a long time before the disposal system and the wasteline were completed and the alterations finished. Have been working indoors and outdoors and now have the satisfaction of leaving the place in good condition. Wish you could see it. There has been no time for guests, too much work.

While in California, Signe used the address of the Rehabilitation Center of San Francicso, 1680 Mission Street. Signe's personal "curriculum vitae" lists participation in a Prosthetic Devices Research Study conducted at the University of California in 1946 and 1947. (Reference is made to the study, sponsored by the National Research Council's Advisory Committee on Artificial Limbs, in Signe's first book, *Training of The Lower Extremity Amputee*, published by Charles C Thomas, 1956.) During this time, she also wrote an article, *Walking Training of the Amputee: Some Biomechanical Considerations,* which appeared in *Physiotherapy Review* (Vol. 27, No. 3), in 1947.

Taking advantage of being in California, Signe attended the national meeting of the American Physical Therapy Association held at Asilomar. Mary Eleanor Brown recalled meeting her at the conference:

> In 1947, a very healthy and exuberant Signe gave me a big hug at the conference. We were on the same program and were put in the same room! It was a grand reunion.

In the fall of 1947, Signe was back in New York. She obtained a position as a research physical therapist at the New York University Institute of Rehabilitation Medicine.

According to Jack Hofkosh, Director of Physical Therapy, Signe's research was involved with the development of the quadrilateral socket and she worked with the physical therapy and prosthetic departments.

If the research role was not enough, Signe also taught Gross Anatomy and Neuroanatomy at Columbia University. That activity is best described by Marie-Louise Franciscus, OTR, of North Fort Meyers, Florida, Professor Emeritus of Columbia University:

> I first met Signe in 1947 when I joined the faculty of Columbia University's College of Physicians and Surgeons as the Associate Director of Occupational Therapy. Signe was doing dissection as she researched muscle-nerve function with Dr. Herbert Elftman, a noted functional anatomist on the Columbia faculty. I had just completed a similar, but far less sophisticated, project with Dr. Linden Edwards at Ohio State University. Signe and I compared notes on several occasions during those early years. Later, with Dr. Elftman teaching anatomy and Signe, kinesiology, a well coordinated and integrated sequence of learning was offered to our OT and PT students. It was during those years that Signe was also working out treatment theories with hemiplegia patients at the Institute for Rehabilitation Medicine. In those days, Signe was indefatigable, a dynamo of energy, moving with such speed from one thing to another that we fondly nicknamed her "The White Tornado" or "The Whirling Dervish."
>
> When she came into our central office, her presence commanded respect and attention. Her quick, incisive mind, her storehouse of knowledge and understanding, and her skill in sharing combined to make her a teacher par excellence.

Signe's interest in promoting good health through exercise brought her back to the Metropolitan Life Insurance Company. The records show that on December 2, 1947, she was reappointed as "the Physical Training Instructress—part time, $20 Tuesday and Thursday PM. No credit allowed for previous employment.''

Despite a very busy work schedule throughout 1948, Signe found peace and quiet when in her home on Bullet Hole Road. Much of her effort was given to planning another small house on the property. She also devoted time to organizing some research material and scientific papers. A little time was allowed to occasionally entertain friends. If it was not for a former Navy ''buddy'', Occupational Therapist Lucy Gore Stead, and her husband Gordon, Signe probably would have spent her fiftieth birthday and New Year's Eve, 1949, all by herself. Lucy and Gordon were on their way to England and stopped in Carmel, New York, to spend the holiday. Signe tried out her new skis, as there was plenty of snow in the pasture around her home. After the refreshing outdoors, it was dinner at the Carmel Country Club. Just before mid-night, they all sat around a small TV (one of the early sets) to wish in the new year of 1949.

Signe started the year with a trip to Chicago and then to San Francisco to participate in a conference on clinical services for amputees, sponsored by the Veterans Administration. She also met with several physicians, some of her physical therapy friends such as Hazel Furscott and Alice Seligman, and had dinner with Bob and Fran Teckemeyer in Santa Rosa. After a day at Mare Island, it was a night plane to New York on January 15. During her brief absence, the cinder-block foundation of the main house was started on her property. Over the next several weeks, while Signe painted basement frames, carpenters were brought in to place the studs. Signe's notes indicate, ''On January 31, decided on a roof instead of a deck over the garage.'' During the construction of the new house, which would take more than two years, Signe lived in the converted old ''chicken coop.''

Another important phase of Signe's life was set into motion with a phone call on February 10, 1949, from Dr. Kessler. Recalling his experiences with Signe at Mare Island, Kessler offered her a full-time job at his Institute in East Orange, New Jersey. Deciding against full time, on

March 1, 1949, she started to work with Kessler three days a week: Tuesday, Wednesday and Thursday. She devoted Tuesday and Thursday late afternoons to Metropolitan Life.

The position at the Institute allowed Signe to further her interest and work with stroke patients. At the Institute in 1949, she first started to use associated reactions and a synergy approach, while simultaneously searching medical literature for information. Her first background publications dealt with the work of Magnus de Kleijn and Simons, translated from publications in German. The methods set forth in Signe's major text, *Movement Therapy in Hemiplegia,* developed gradually thereafter during clinical practice.

The abstract of ''Haltung,'' chapter 111 of Magnus' book *KORPERSTELLUNG* (Body Posture), appeared in the Physical Therapy Review (33:281–282, June 1953). The abstract of A. Simon's article, *KOPFHALTUNG UND MUSKELTONUS* (Head Posture and Muscle Tone), was printed in the Physical Therapy Review (33:409–419, August,1953).

A slight change in routine and enjoyment occurred on March 25 with a renewal in family ties, when her Mother and older sister Elsa arrived from Sweden. Signe took great pride in sharing her little piece of country life with them.

Work was a priority for Signe. She persevered and devoted just about all of her time to her many professional activities. According to her notes, there were no further entries until November, 1949, when she had a visit from two United Nations representatives from Egypt. In mid-November, Signe's life was centered around ''much work at K.I. and in building Hill House.''

Signe's notes for 1949 end with ''wishing you a thrifty 1950.'' The new year started off with a generous offer made by Signe to two special friends on January 28–29: ''Elizabeth and Ben Combs had honeymoon at Hill House, not as yet fully finished.''

Despite maintaining an exceptionally tight working schedule, Signe embarked on another major project in the Spring of 1950 that eventually would lead to her first major published book. At the Kessler Institute she worked with Donald Kerr. He was to be her future collaborator on a special text related to the care of the amputee. Signe's experiences at Mare Island with the Navy made her an "expert" in rehabilitation of the lower extremity amputee. She relished the opportunity to share her research and findings related to amputees, but did not realize how much time this project would take or what frustrations would lie ahead.

Kerr was a graduate of Tulane, Class of 1935. As an amputee, he became a champion badminton player and an outstanding all-around athlete. Kerr demonstrated how capable an amputee could be and served as a role model and inspiration to many disabled people. Between 1944 and 1947, he was a consultant to the American Red Cross, working with the Surgeons-General of the Army and Navy. He proposed plans for special rehab wards at Mare Island. From 1948 to 1950, he was in charge of amputee training at K.I. and later became Director of the National Institute for Amputee Rehabilitation. Don and Signe became very close and often traveled together to promote amputee training. They made three trips around the country, applying their approach to amputee training. In an August 9, 1986, phone conversation, Don said: "Signe taught me anatomy. She always shared and wanted to help others. She could get things done that were important."

One particular demonstration was vividly recalled by Herb Jones, PT, now living in Miami. In 1949 and 1950, he was a therapist at the State of Connecticut Veterans Hospital. At the facility, he was involved in a program in prosthetics to help many of the veterans who had become amputees. In an August 10, 1986 letter, Herb describes the situation:

> We arranged for Signe and the VA team to include Rocky Hill on the schedule. Signe did her usual excellent presentation to the staff and with her was Don Kerr. Don was not a veteran but a man who lost one lower limb (AK) when he was young and had rehabilitated himself with a prosthesis. He played badminton, tennis, baseball and football.
>
> Donald's favorite stunt was to jump up on a table or desk and then jump off, landing on his prosthesis, (then

only single axis knees were available). As part of the program, he did this in front of the group of old men we were trying to motivate to walk with walkers. When they saw Don's activities, most of the patients started to wheel out of the room—yelling 'you're not going to get me to do that stuff.' Signe was upset with Don as well as the patients. She felt such a demonstration scared the patients, even the younger one. She went around trying to explain to the men that we wouldn't expect them to jump off the table but that Don did that to show there are no limitations to what can be done. She saved the day and we were able to go on and develop a very good amputee program.

Signe was named the Director of Professional Education at the Institute. By April, 1950, she and Don had an outline for an amputee manual. Many hours were spent in discussion of content, preparing drawings of stick figures, and writing and rewriting material. Unfortunately, the amputee manual was to take much of Signe's time. Having a collaborator brought on some very special problems including disagreements on the material. It would take five years of intermittent work to see the manuscript completed. For compulsive Signe, this was a disappointment.

To demonstrate the type of work schedule Signe maintained, one need only look at her 1950 appointment book:

4/7: visit from Donald Kerr and Pat, we worked on Amputee Manual.

4/22: Amputee conference, K.I.

5/1: First day of Amputee conference in Toronto. Leave of absence without pay from K.I. and Met Life.

5/1–4: Visited Lyndhurst Lodge also Workmen's Compensation Hospital and Rehab Center outside Toronto. Then returned by plane to N.Y.

5/13: to Philadelphia meeting of American College of Surgeons, Committee on Training with John Seeley and Donald Kerr.

5/22: wrote foreword to amputee manual.

5/25:	by plane to Memphis to lecture at Association for Physical Medicine & Rehab, Hotel Peabody, dinner in Mississippi with Dr. J. Young and Dr. F. Mahoney.
5/27:	back to N.Y.
5/29:	started chapter for Dr. Bierman's book.
6/5:	back to work at K.I.
8/21:	meeting with Page and Reilly re division of work, job analysis.
9/11:	conference with Mr. Miller, Near East Foundation.
9/18:	plane to Pittsburgh, Mellon Institute
9/21:	visit to D.T. Watson Home, Leetsdale
9/22:	Lecture at Mellon Institute on "Training in the Use of Braces."
10/14:	Visit from Art and Helen Brown
10/15:	Visit from Donald Kerr
10/18:	met Donald at Mahopac Airport. Plane trip over Mahopac, Carmel, Bullet Hole, etc.

The next notation had great significance. On October 19, Signe went to the Greek Consulate to obtain a visa. She also sent a foot locker off to Greece. Less than a month before, Signe had met with a Mr. Miller of the Near East Foundation. It was at that meeting Signe decided to undertake an important assignment in Greece which would involve her setting up a rehabilitation program. It was not a spur-of-the-moment decision. The plan was initiated in the spring of 1950, culminating with Signe being named a Fulbright Scholar! A letter of June 9 from Gordon T. Bowles, Executive Secretary of the Conference Board of Associated Research Council, Committee on International Exchange of Persons, to Mildred Elson, Executive Secretary of the APTA requested a reference on Signe. The Committee was prepared to support a physical therapist for a year's assignment in Greece. Bowles indicated the grant would allow "Miss Signe Brunnstrom to be a Visiting Lecturer in Physical Therapy in Greece." As such, she would be allowed to "teach any or all aspects of rehabilitation of an orthopedic and neurological nature." Mildred Elson responded on June 12:

> Miss Brunstromm is, in my opinion, eminently qualified as a Visiting Lecturer in Greece. She has the basic knowledge and clinical experience in both orthopedic and neurological conditions to teach all aspects of rehabilitation in this country or in any foreign country. She has shared her knowledge through articles in the Physical Therapy review and prepared a movie ''Peripheral Nerve Injuries'' which the American Physical Therapy Association copied and loaned to schools of physical therapy and groups of members. Miss Brunnstrom enjoys the highest respect both personally and professionally of her colleagues.She is energetic with possible excess of nervous energy. She is inclined to drive herself too hard. She will always give more to her work than is normally demanded.

Further correspondence to the Near East Foundation from E. Jane Carlin, Educational Consultant for the APTA stated:

> Miss Brunnstrom has published many scientific papers relating to physical therapy. She was also responsible for the preparation of a film on peripheral nerve injuries which has had wide circulation. Her references and reputation, both personally and professionally are outstanding.

Before finalizing the assignment, Signe contacted Helen Kaiser, Associate in Physical Therapy, in charge of the Division of Physical Therapy at Duke University in Durham, North Carolina. Helen had organized a program in physical therapy in Athens in 1946 that had little on-going success after her return to the states. Helen was very pleased that Signe was chosen for the challenging task of re-establishing a rehabilitation program in Athens. In a letter of August 11, 1950, Helen wrote Signe:

> I am so glad it is you who are going to Greece. I have been so worried that they would settle on someone who is merely travel minded and would not take the assignment seriously. It is a difficult one; one that

will require infinite patience and perseverance. But I am sure that you will find it worth the effort.

When you come to understand their ways, and do not expect them to function as we do, you will find the Greeks a delightful people with whom to work.

Helen offered Signe some pertinent information and advice related to orthopedists, surgeons, medicine in general and the social and political situation as she observed it in 1946:

I would say that you must be extremely wary as to where and with whom you make your first contacts and affiliations. The political situation is complicated. The Greeks are very wily and know no ethics such as we recognize in this country. I do not say this in any sense of criticism, for their economic and social situation is entirely different from this country, but one must understand it before one can move forward with any degree of wisdom. The Near East Foundation can help you tremendously in the political aspects, but they are babes in the woods when it comes to medicine. (Helen Kaiser died September 8,1988.)

The assignment to Greece did not come as a surprise to Signe's co-workers at K.I. Dr. Kessler himself had a hand in the plan. In his book, *The Knife is Not Enough,* Kessler mentions that he visited Greece as the President of the International Society for the Welfare of Cripples. The Hellenic Society for Crippled Children sought assistance in developing a program for training physical therapists and he sent "Miss Signe Brunnstrom, chief physical therapist of the Kessler Institute, to Athens to assist the Hellenic Society and to establish a much needed school for physical therapists."

On October 22, 1950, a limousine picked Signe up at Bullet Hole and drove her to what was then called Idlewild Airport. The staff of the Kessler Institute was at the airport to see her off.

The British Overseas Air Line Stratocruiser landed in London and the next day Signe was on a British-European

Airways flight to France. Ever exuberant about travel, Signe offered a detailed description about the trip and her first week in Athens:

> Departure from London, BEA over France, stop at Nice, overnight in Rome. Flight Rome-Athens along coast—Vesuvius—island of Elba, Napoleon's exile—over "M-P joints" and "heel" of Italy—Ionean Sea—island of Corfu—Bay of Corinth—Isthmus of Corinth, 4 to 8 miles wide, transversed by canal. From the air, Greece looks like a contour map (plane goes low enough to give this impression). It is very mountainous. On the mainland to the left snowcapped mountains—among them Parnassus, the dwelling of the Gods, and Helicon, the abode of the Muses. To the right the mountain on the Peloponnesus, also snow covered. Plane crosses over Piraeus, the harbor of Athens, connected with Athens by an electric train; circles the airport, at which time a beautiful view of Athens is obtained; Acropolis on a hill overlooking the city, on top of which there is a small chapel. Airport near the sea. Southern sun and clear skies—mountains in the background—blue Aegean Sea. Met by foreign director of Near East Foundation, a Fulbright dietitian and Mr. and Mrs. Poulopoulus.

She stayed at the King George Hotel on Syntagma Square. It was very modern with a private bath. The cost with dinner and "petit dejeuner" came to almost $10. The next day, October 26, Signe went to the fashionable tennis club for lunch. She walked along the Royal Gardens and past the Temple of Zeus. At the club she lunched with Mr. Hill of the Near East Foundation and met several important people including representatives from the Ministry of Health, a Professor of Orthopedics and the director of the Educational Foundation. In her own words, Signe said: " . . . felt enthused about all I was going to do and the friendly reception." That evening she had dinner with a Greek family, friends of Mr. and Mrs. Poulopoulus.

October 28 is a special holiday in Greece. Signe enjoyed all the events of the day and wrote descriptive notes of the occasion:

> Three holidays in memory of October 28, 1940 when Metaxa said "NO" to Italian demands of jurisdiction over Epirus and establishment of military bases in Greece. At sunrise and sundown 21 gun salute; streets stirred with uniformed men and civilians: military bands marched through the streets, patriotic songs heard; at 10 a.m. Royal Family rode through streets to church service in cathedral; then to Parliament building where, in front of the tomb of the Unknown Soldier, the King reviewed the troops; Royal car preceded by a guard of 35 men on white horses; the same number on brown horses followed; streets lined with Army and Navy guard; civilians 10 persons deep or more along the streets, every half hour a ceremonial changing of the guards took place in front of the tomb; special guard in colorful costume (white long stockings, short kilt, shoes with long bent up pointed toes, pompons, red head gear); troop review lasted two hours. First came disabled veterans in wheelchairs pushed by nurses (decided the next OXI day the veterans were going to push their own); Greek troops march with precision, swinging the arm opposite the rifle in an exaggerated forward-backward swing, but no goose stepping; except for characteristic marching it could have been American troops (all material, uniforms, etc., comes from the States), infantry, motorized cavalry, artillery, tanks, engineering troops, hospital units; Navy parade; Air Force in sky forming letters OXI, roaring over city time after time in perfect formation.

While in Greece, Signe wanted to live in Kifissia, but the Near East Foundation director insisted she take a vacant room in the NEF apartment at the corner of Jan Smuts and Valeoritou Street. Signe was upset with that decision, as the area was the noisiest part of the city, had a strong smell of gas due to all of the cars, and the plumbing was poor. Unhappy with this situation, she looked into finding another apartment and was upset to see the prices demanded of Americans. For a two-room apartment in the city, well-furnished but dark, the cost was $175 a month. She also saw an apartment with no kitchen, hardly any furniture and a bathroom to share. For Greek persons, Signe was told the cost would be 600,000 drachmas. But for an American, one million!

Another disappointment was the cost of food and supplies. Signe noted that a roll of toilet paper cost a dollar; a box of tissues almost two dollars; a jar of marmalade one dollar; and nylon hose six to eight dollars. A cup of coffee cost three times as much as a small glass of wine, "the latter 500 drachmas or 3 ⅓ cents."

Within two weeks of arriving in Athens, Signe wrote Mildred Elson at the APTA in New York City that she was "in the middle of a rather ticklish situation." A law had been drafted by the Ministry of Health to provide the legal background for establishment of a physical therapy school and regulation of the practice. The proposed law would give a license to practice physical therapy only to graduates of the new school. Signe wanted to insert a clause to provide for reciprocity with schools in other countries having the same standards. A major problem was that she could not be certain if the Greek school would reach the standards set for similar programs in the United States or in most of the European countries. In the letter to Mildred Elson, Signe indicated she thought some kind of reciprocity was being contemplated and she would like to pave the way for an eventual inclusion of Greece "in the family of physical therapy nations."

Mildred Elson responded to Signe in a letter of November 7 indicating there was no reciprocity between any of the countries that Signe mentioned. She recognized that standards differed from country to country. Her suggestion to Signe was to have a statement included in the new law indicating that "those qualified and holding a certificate in their own country could be permitted to practice providing that all certificates of education and employment are reviewed by the Ministry and are found to be authentic and are the equivalent of the requirements of the Ministry.'' Ms. Elson concluded her letter with the statement, ''I'm not sure I've helped you very much since writing things into law makes them awfully final.''

Throughout November and December Signe made many contacts with personnel in the School of Nursing at Evangelismos Hospital, the military limb shop, the People's hospital, Children's Hospital, the Ministry of Health, military hospitals, and other facilities serving the disabled. She was convinced that there was a most pressing need for rehabilitation services (especially for amputees) and for the training of physical therapists. What she found were a variety of agencies devoted to their own interests with little support for administering the agencies to meet the needs of the disabled. During her visits she saw severe overcrowding, no facilities for rehabilitation, no physical or occupational therapy, a lot of American equipment not in use, and minimal training for nurses in the care of paraplegics and amputees. All of this made it imperative that the school for physical therapists be established, but Signe ran into many obstacles. In addition, if there was to be a new program, it would have to meet Signe's standards. Personnel of the Near East Foundation pressed to have the school program start in the spring of 1951. That gave Signe just three months to put the entire plan together. That is if the government approved the plan and passed the new law. In a letter of November 6 to Dr. Kessler, she wrote:

> My work here is progressing along two lines, indicated by my official titles, namely: ''Fulbright Director, School of Physical Therapy, University of Athens,'' and ''Near East Foundation Advisor in Rehabilitation.'' As to the first of my jobs, we are still in the process of drawing up legislation, which has to go through the Ministry of Public Health and then the Ministry of Finances before it goes to the legislature. I have had several meetings at the Ministry, and with good luck the law may be passed in a month from now, but it may

> also take considerably longer. I cannot select any students for the PT classes until the law is passed, but I am doing preparatory work on curriculum, teaching material, etc. The school is to be connected with one of the larger hospitals, but it is not even decided which one. There are a great many complications due to politics and the instability of the government has its repercussions on everything regulated by the Ministries.

Referring to her second title, Signe mentioned she had "80 to 100 leg amputees at the Psychico Amputation Hostel." She suggested that Donald Kerr would be a most welcomed staff member who could organize the hostel. Describing rounds with the director of the hostel, she wrote:

> I never in my life saw so many strange looking stumps. The 'sites of election' is either an unknown term to Greek physicians or they don't believe in them. In many BK stumps the fibula was longer than the tibia, but strangely enough there were no abrasions, although many of the amputees have been wearing peglegs or other types of self-made legs for years. I am starting a general conditioning program in each dormitory until the Nisson hut is ready for the training program and I am covering one dormitory (about 20 beds) each day until I have been through the five dormitories. Everybody is just as helpful as they can be, and the amputees who got no attention today were asking when they could start? Hope that this enthusiasm lasts.

Summing up her concern for the amputees, Signe recalled that the main purpose of her presence in Athens was to start the PT school: " . . . and as soon as the preliminary (legislative) phase is past, I will devote all my time to the school." With less than three months in Greece, Signe's frustration with the lack of movement by the authorities was evident.

To start the new year of 1951, Signe prepared a memo January 9 to Mr. Archer, the Foreign Director of the N.E.F. It clearly spelled out her concerns and plan:

> From previous memos and conversations you are aware of my opinion in regard to the inadvisability of starting physical therapy instruction in the spring or early summer. I have discussed this matter with several other people who know Greek conditions and find that they agree with me. Here are some of the reasons:
>
> 1. Didactic instruction should more or less follow the University schedule, that is, start in the Fall. Clinical practice may continue through the summer months after one year of instruction but obviously should not precede theoretic instruction.
> 2. High school spring graduates must be given a chance to apply for the three year course. The same would apply to physical education instructors who are now employed and of 1951 graduates of the Academy of Physical Education who would qualify for the 1 year course. Note that the 1951 graduating class is unusually large and that only a very small number of the graduates have a chance to be employed.
> 3. A considerable amount of time must elapse between the printing of the government decree and the closing time for applications in order to make proper selection of students.
> 4. It is undesirable to have a change of director and instructor after two or three months.
> 5. Starting an intensive course of instruction during the hot summer months will not appeal neither to instructors or to students.

Added to this memo was a concluding paragraph that must have been a "bombshell" to the foundation. Signe put the ultimatum in writing:

> For me to remain in Athens for a period of nine months would serve no useful purpose. I am, therefore, applying to the Educational Foundation for a shortening of my Fulbright award from nine months to five months. If my application is approved my term would be up on March 23rd. If by that time I have not com-

pleted the course for amputee instructors which is expected to begin without delay, I am willing to stay over without remuneration for a short additional period. Another reason for my wishing to have the Fulbright award discontinued is of a financial nature. The funds which I am now in the process of having transferred from Sweden to the States will help me meet my financial obligations in the States for about three more months. I can under no circumstances afford a longer stay in Athens. The acceptance of Fulbright remuneration for five months when Drachmas cannot be exchanged into dollars means an outright financial loss of $1,000 to me. This matter, again, needs no detailed explanations since I have discussed it with you on previous occasions.

Two days later on January 11, Signe sent a memo to the Chairman and members of the Rehabilitation Committee in reference to the Physical Therapy School. She reminded the group that she was sent to Athens under the Fulbright 1950–51 program as a visiting lecturer to organize instruction and to teach in a school of physical therapy under the auspices of the Greek government. She stated:

> It is unfortunate indeed that nearly three months have elapsed since my arrival and that the legislation which must precede the beginning of the school has not as yet been passed, Furthermore, after the passage of the law, a minimum of two or three additional months will be required before instruction can actually begin. The Government decree must be printed, the Administrative committee of the school be appointed and start functioning, application blanks be sent to prospective students, applications filed, students selected, etc. Even if the progress of the law is from now on more rapid than it has been in the past, it would be late spring or early summer before instruction could begin.

Signe then suggested that the preliminaries for the establishment of the school be continued, but that the beginning of the school term be set for September. By that time another American specialist could be engaged to carry on the work. She also indicated that an American specialist need not be present for the entire preliminary period. The memo concluded with Signe's comments about shortening of her stay and her concern for how money was being spent:

> The spending of Fulbright funds is not justified unless a positive benefit can be derived from it. Likewise, my personal financial sacrifices, which are considerable, seem useless unless I make a definite contribution.

A few days later, January 16, Signe had a memo prepared to be sent to all the directors of physical therapy programs and schools in the States. She appealed to the directors to try to find a qualified individual who would be interested in accepting the terms of a Fulbright grant so that the original work done by Helen Kaiser in 1946 could be rekindled. It was evident that Signe had definitely decided to leave in the spring without waiting for a replacement.

In the meanwhile, Signe changed her living quarters, which brought some pleasure by getting her out of the downtown area.

In a letter of March 11 (1951) to her dear American friend Margit Aden, Signe wrote:

> The furnished room at Valeoritou Street, misnamed, "personnel house" was a rather gloomy experience. The N.E.F. maintains the apartment partly for an office for the blind, partly for two employees (an American nurse and a dietitian,) who have been in the employ of the Foundation for many years. For two old maids to have another old maid walking in on them at the wish of the NEF director, was not a happy event. I would never have rented that gloomy room had it not been that the foreign director insisted that I take it. I kept it for four months, then I moved out. Now I have a lovely sunny room with a balcony at Kifissia, a summer resort place about half an hour by bus from the center of Ath-

ens. I am enjoying the fresh air, the sun and my freedom in general. To my surprise I find that it is not any more expensive than the other place, where I got soaked on a lot of extras, such as heat, electricity, water, soap, toilet paper, maid service, etc. Here I pay 30,000 drachmas a day which includes breakfast. That certainly is reasonable for a first class hotel. Compare it with the other place where they charged me 15,000 for coffee and toast in the morning (imagine $1.00) just for coffee and miserable toast, no marmalade, and you could see that I should have made the change a long time ago.

As noted, Signe was not able to transfer her funds out of Greece. Once again she demonstrated her generosity by inviting some relatives to vacation in Greece as her guests. She mentioned their forthcoming visit in a March 11 letter to Margit Aden:

> My brothers-in-law and two of my nieces are coming to Greece to help me spend my surplus drachmas, so I guess there will be no unused money by April 11. None of my sisters could come.

In another letter to Margit on April 10, Signe mentions the surplus drachmas again:

> My brother-in-law from Stockholm and my two nieces from Skane have been here close to three weeks to help me spend my leftover drachmas. They melted away rapidly, some ten millions in three weeks, but I still have more of the darned stuff left which I don't know what to do with. A queer predicament.

One troublesome point did develop regarding the funds. Signe was required to pay U.S. income taxes on the monies paid through the Fulbright award, even though she could not place the funds in her American account. She was very annoyed with the American tax system in that regard.

While she continued planning the new school program, Signe also carefully watched the lack of progress of the necessary legislation. She completed her survey on rehabilitation needs noting that the most pressing requirements were for services for paraplegics and amputees. She wanted an Administrative Committee appointed for the school. "Greeks will not work as long as Americans work," she stated in her notes. Later only one month before she left, a temporary committee was set up.

Signe made her plans to leave Greece in April. She wrote Margit Aden on March 11:

> Luckily I have been able to shorten my Fulbright contract from 9 to 5 months, so my term here will officially be up on March 23rd, and I will wind up my work by April 11, when I am leaving for Munich, where I will stay two days, then a week in England, and if all goes well, I will be back in the States on April 29th.

Concern for Signe's departure reached the Ministry of Social Welfare. On March 17, Secretary General M. P. Goutos wrote:

> I am sincerely sorry that you are leaving on April the 10th. My government and I will be only too willing to do all that is necessary so that you can stay a little longer in Athens, because we believe that the services you rendered to our country are the most useful ones under the present circumstances, even more so than any other services rendered by other foreign specialists who remained in this country for a short while. I personally regret that the Greek bureaucracy didn't help you enough.

Evidently, it was not just frustrations with the system and lack of progress on developing the school that precipitated Signe's decision to leave Greece. Signe had major concerns about finances and her home on Bullet Hole Road. The March 11 letter to Margit described her overall financial problem:

> My agonies in regard to the Bullet Hole, which have been the worst part of my stay here, will soon be over. If I had been able to rent the Hill House, or if I had been smart enough to get a real caretaker for the place, I would probably have stayed my term out here. There is so much to do in rehabilitation, that I feel a little bit bad about leaving, but financially, I am now so bad off that I cannot afford to stay any longer. Fortunately, I have been able to transfer a small sum of money from Sweden to the States in order to keep up my FHA payments, insurance and taxes. Immediately when I get home, I will get busy and try to rent both the Hill House and the summer house, which, if I succeed, should somewhat better my finances.

In addition to her concerns relating to financial problems, Signe was in real distress. She actually was quite physically ill. A description of her illness was included in a letter to Margit on April 3:

> I may have sounded low in some of my letters. The fact is that I have been more or less ill since January. I was in bed with the ''flu'' whatever that is and I got a series of penicillin shots, since the doctor thought it might develop into pneumonia. The week thereafter I had to be up to give a public lecture which had been advertised widely with special printed invitations and much fuss, and I have been struggling ever since with a rise in temperature in the evenings, chills and a terrific cough. I got a second series of x-rays, blood counts, sputum examinations, and then streptomyecin. Still the cough goes on. My productive capacity is only about half of normal. I am just hanging on this week to finish the course, but I am like a rag. A strange sensation when you are not used to it. I am looking forward to a long rest at the Bullet Hole. As long as the x-ray is negative for TB, I think the Bullet Hole will lick the germs.

On April 6, Signe graduated her first amputee instructor class. That same morning she had chest x-rays taken. She described the situation:

> All was not well with my one lung. The Naval doctor who re-examined me wanted me admitted to the hospital right away. So here I am (April 10) in the Evangelismos Hospital, American Wing, run by Navy doctors. I am very well taken care of and have been in bed for four days. The doctors expect it to take some time to make a differential diagnosis. There are all kinds of ugly possibilities. I have myself picked "atypical virus pneumonia" as the most attractive of the possible diagnoses. I probably had pneumonia in January, at the time unrecognized, and I have had it ever since. Excessive work or a hike in the country would bring about a raise in temperature. A day in bed, and the temperature would go down, but the strange crowded burning feeling in my chest remained. TB is not yet completely ruled out, but it is less probable. Tests and more x-rays will have to be taken.
>
> In the meantime, I have had a wonderful rest on the first good bed I have run across in Greece, resting my head on a real pillow instead of the sandbaglike monsters which the hotels offer you. Besides vitamin pills, 6-hourly shots of streptomyecin, and "postural drainage," my treatment also consists of delicious meals, milk, butter, and American coffee, all of which I have been doing without for the last six months. The cook here is a Greek who used to work at the Waldorf Astoria, so you may realize that there is no better place to be ill than in this American Wing.

The doctors suggested that Signe would have to stay at the hospital two to three weeks and then rest for another three weeks. She had to change all of her plans for Munich and England. In addition, she canceled an audience with the Queen of Greece and a lecture in Rome. After more tests were conducted, the doctors advised Signe that she probably would be discharged around April 23, but they advised her to check into a medical center as soon as possible upon her return to the States. On April 26, a tired, ill and frustrated Signe Brunnstrom left Athens and headed home. In her notes titled "Six Months in Greece," she summed up her feelings:

> Standard of Behavior of Greeks:
> Promise you everything under the sun, but have no intention of keeping promises—is a way of speaking and should not be regarded as not keeping a promise. Greeks do not like to work; poor pay in Civil Service jobs; graft; dependence upon American work and financial aid; politics; constant change in government changed 6 times in recent years. After last elections Prime Minister, Field Marshal Alexander Papagos, Greek Conservative Party, promises a house cleaning. "It is wrong to expect everything from U.S.A."Regretted leaving; learned to love the country and the people in spite of all their shortcomings; feeling of futility, situation very difficult; Greeks will do very little if anything as long as the Americans are there; but, if American assistance is withdrawn, in the words of a Greek, "that will be the end of Greece."

In a lengthy article, *Amputee Training in Greece,* prepared by Signe and published in the October, 1951 Physical Therapy Review, she wrote:

> Rehabilitation of all types of disabled persons is urgently needed in Greece. Seeing the amount of work which should be done and having to proceed so slowly on all fronts is a frustrating experience. The physical therapy school could not get underway because of a legislative hold-up, but, at least in the field of amputee rehabilitation, something was achieved. It was a drop in the bucket, to be sure, but even a small amount of success makes you rejoice when you worked so hard for it.

Dr. Kessler in his 1968 book, refers to the problem Signe had in trying to establish a physical therapy school:

> Miss Brunnstrom stayed in Athens for a year, but it was a year of disappointment and frustration. The local physicians apparently were so fearful of competition from any new professional group that they thwarted all efforts to start the school. Subsequently we sent another physical therapist from the States, but opposition was too strong and his efforts also proved to be in vain.

Ironically, despite all of Signe's efforts to initiate rehabilitation activities, little remains of her work. In searching for information about her six months in Greece, I corresponded with the Executive Director of the United States Educational Foundation in Greece, The Fulbright Program. In a response to the inquiry, William R. Ammerman wrote on August 8, 1984:

> Our records show that Ms. Brunnstrom was a Fulbrighter in Athens during the 1950–51 academic year. Specifically, she lectured at the University of Athens from October 1950–April 1951. The only note I can find indicates that Ms. Brunnstrom lectured in Physical Therapy at the University. Unfortunately, I do not know anyone who might remember Ms. Brunnstrom's work. The only record we have is a small index card which we keep on all grantees with only the bare outlines of the assignment.

Signe's expertise in rehabilitation was always in demand. She could be employed in many situations. Why then, did she decide to become a Fulbright lecturer and go to Greece? Her friend, Margit, in correspondence with Signe, suggested it was an "escape" from her responsibilities in the States. Signe had her own reasons and explanation for taking on the demanding role in Greece. She replied to Margit's comments in a letter of April 3:

> The "escape" as you call it can also be given more appropriate names. If you get into an unbearable situation at the place where you work and still feel that the

place offers too much on the positive side to give it up, the only sensible thing is to get away for a while to get perspective. My trip to Greece has served that purpose very well.

My other reason for wanting to go to Greece was that it was a challenge to me. I somehow knew that this was a job which was very much needed. This will sound silly to you, but have you ever had a feeling of responsibility toward the world? You won't believe it, but after having heard about the Greek deal, I would have had a feeling of guilt had I allowed my desire for comfortable living and my love of the Bullet Hole to prevent me from going. I guess it was something like deciding to go into the service during the war.

Thirdly, I guess I still have something of an adventurer in me. It was too good an opportunity to miss, a new country, a new language, the tales of antiquity to verify, the beautiful Greek landscape to discover, a sniff of European air to mix with the Main Street atmosphere of West Orange, N.J. The fact that I couldn't do the job which I came here to do was a great disappointment to me and it spoiled my fun here for a considerable time. Now that I practically completed a course for amputee instructors of 8 weeks duration against formidable odds I feel very pleased with myself. I realize now that I felt I could and should move a mountain, but that was really quite impossible. Hence, I must be satisfied at having loosened a few slates from the mountainside, and that I have done.

My stay in Greece has brought a lot of headaches, but also a lot of pleasure. Now that it is done, I wouldn't have it undone for anything.

Signe paid quite a price for her devotion to duty in Greece. On April 29, 1951, looking far-older than her 53 years, she arrived at Idlewild Airport in New York and was met by Dr. Kessler, Genevieve Reilly and Bill Page. She was driven directly to her Bullet Hole home by Page. Three days later she saw a Dr. Leff in Newark, and had x-rays and a thoroscope. The once super-dynamic, enthusiastic and energetic Signe received doctor's orders: ''to rest to heal the spot on lung.''

Chapter Five

The Author

During her forced "rest period" in the spring of 1951, Signe prepared the article on the rehabilitation situation in Greece referred to in the previous chapter. She did not remain idle for very long. With the new experiences gained in working with the Greek amputees, she also went back to preparing material for the amputee manual. Her notes indicate, "February-March, manuscript work throughout both months." She also worked on the grounds around her home, rented the upper level of her Hill House, "shot a woodchuck in the vegetable garden" and slowly recuperated. With the rest, her physician told her the spot was normal.

On May 20, Dr. Kessler visited Signe at Bullet Hole. He offered her an opportunity to return to the institute in East Orange as a physical therapy consultant. Signe noted the visit with the comment, "He was anxious to have me again." Less than two months later, she was back at work at the institute. Included in the business of the day on her return was playing host to a visiting group of German professionals, Signe spoke fluent German.

About six months before Signe returned to the institute, Ruth Dickinson accepted a P.T. staff position at the facility. Ruth was well aware of Signe's work in the navy and her reputation as an outstanding therapist. Among the first activities Signe undertook at the institute was to set up a series of amputee conferences. Ruth was there, and she recalled, "I lucked out! What an education I had!" Ruth's responsibilities included taking copious notes about everything that was presented at the conferences. This included the surgical procedures, the prosthetic selection, the pre-prosthetic and prosthetic training. For Ruth, "the highlight, of course, was Signe's presentation. Her enthusiasm, the clarity of her lectures, her respect, kindness, and concern for patients who demonstrated their skills, her clinical expertise and her professionalism—all were an inspiration." Ruth also saw some humor in Signe's demonstrations, "especially when she would illustrate what happened when her 'vertical projection of the center of gravity fell outside her base of support'. She would almost topple over, quickly regain her balance all the while talking animatedly about prosthetic training techniques." There were many proud moments enjoyed by Ruth as she began to assist Signe with some of the patient demonstrations.

Anyone who knew Signe well was aware of her love for animals. Reminiscing about her early childhood, Ingegerd spoke about the family's dog, "Hey", who once bit a man "because he looked like a bad person." Signe loved dogs and horses. In 1953, she picked up a stray dog that could only be classified as a "mutt." Signe named her "Kaya" which is Swedish for blackbird. She was to be Signe's constant companion at Bullet Hole. Kaya had eight puppies on November 9, 1955. Signe decided to keep one male, who was named "Rebel". Kaya had a long life. She was with Signe for 18 years!

Throughout 1952 and 1953, Signe and Donald continued their collaboration, and work on the manual progressed slowly. During this period, Ruth was privy to Signe's account of the development of the manuscript. She helped with the training programs of most of the amputees photographed for the manual. "Don, himself an amputee," Ruth recollected, "was as intense, knowledgeable and dynamic as Signe. Two 'dynamos', two strong personalities and sometimes two big sparks would fly!"

Regular physical education classes were reinitiated at Metropolitan's gym on January 9, 1953. Signe referred to the classes with the special comment, "started a six week course with music at M.L.I." Apparently, she was well ahead of the modern bio-fitness craze in which music plays such an important part.

A physical therapist friend from Sweden, Agnetta Olsson, arrived in New York to spend some time with Signe. Anxious to show her the Kessler Institute, Signe drove Agnetta there on February 4. She also observed Signe at work during one of her M.L.I. classes in the city. (Several months later, they were to meet again in Philadelphia and travel across the country.)

On March 12, Signe met with Donald Kerr in Lodi, New Jersey, to discuss developing separate publications on amputees. The result of that get-together was a "blow-up" with Donald. By the end of the month, Don returned to Bullet Hole to work with Signe on the prosthetic chapter and material on "walking faults." That was not to be the end of their problems with the manuscript.

Ingegerd returned to the States on June 3 on the S.S. Gripsholm. Signe picked her up at the pier and drove directly to Bullet Hole Road in Carmel. To help with the finances, the house was rented, and three days later they started a fantastic cross-country trip. It was obvious from Signe's notes that the trip was quite extensive. They saw more of the United States than most Americans ever do. Signe loved to travel, and here was an opportunity to show her adopted country to her sister and a friend. The following itinerary is taken directly from Signe's personal notes:

June 7: Agnetta met us in Philadelphia. We saw Independence Hall.

June 8: Pennsylvania Turnpike, Donegal over-night, then Pennsylvania, West Virginia and Ohio. Lewisburg, Ohio, over night near Indiana border.

June 9: Through Indiana "the Hoosier State" and Illinois (Lincoln's homes). Throughout the trip,

	Agnetta and I alternated driving. Hannibal, Missouri over night. Through Missouri, Kansas and into Colorado—493 miles—overnight to Colorado Springs.
June 11:	"Garden of the Gods." Cave Dwellers, Pike's Peak
June 15:	Left Colorado Springs for Glenwood Springs overnight.
June 16:	Horseback riding, State Fish Hatchery, swimming in hot pool, overnight at Green River.
June 18:	Overnight in Afton, Wyoming
June 19:	Arrived in Yellowstone Park.
June 20–22:	Drove around Yellowstone, hiked, saw bears, moose and calf, mule deer, antelope, Drove out West entrance to Tova Falls and overnight at Blackboat.
June 23:	Reno, Nevada, overnight. arrived at Lake Tahoe, stayed at Neilson's place.
June 26:	left Tahoe, via Sacramento to Vallejo
June 29:	to Berkeley. Inge and I had lunch with Professor Eberhart
June 30:	Drove Inge to San Francisco via Golden Gate Bridge.
July 1:	started attending course at Kabat Kaiser Rehab, Vallejo. Agnetta same.
July 5:	to Dillon beach with Maggie Knott, Dorothy Voss and Margery Ionta.

While in California, Signe maintained a very active business and social calendar. She held conferences with various physicians at Kabat-Kaiser Rehab Center. On July 14, it was dinner with her former Navy colleague, Bob Teckemeyer and his wife, Fran. Two days later, Signe participated in a roundtable discussion with Dr. Kabat. On July 18, she visited Shirley and Thomas Mainwaring (Shirley was the X-ray Technician at Mare Island during WW II). On July 19, she spent the day with Lucille Daniels and Marian Williams. While there, she abstracted a German article with Marian.

Francoise Lamote, PT-OT, (now of Ajaccio, France,) in a letter of August 30, 1987, recalled meeting Signe while in California in 1953:

> In 1953, I was a Fulbright student P.T.-O.T. from the University of Southern California. I went to Vallejo to follow the courses of Dr. Kabat (neuro-muscular facilitation). Amongst the young students, I met an elderly PT who was there just as a student to learn what Knott and Voss had to tell. Actually, she knew much more than the teachers who were supposed to teach her. She followed the course as a good learner. It was amazing.

When it was time to go home, it was just Inge and Signe who headed back to New York. Agnetta stayed at Kabat-Kaiser's.

Again Signe kept a detailed travel account of the auto trip. It reads like a Cook's Travelog.

Aug. 12: left Palo Alto, swam in Donner Lake: to Sparks, Nevada.
Aug. 14: Wendover, Nevada, Salt Lake Desert, Utah and Salt lake City. Sightseeing Ft. Badger, lunch in Lyman.
Aug. 15: Rock Springs, Medicine Bow, Cheyenne, Sidney, Ogalla, Nebraska (saw Indians)
Aug. 16: to Odessa (34 inhabitants) by passed Cairo landed in Denison, Iowa.
Aug. 21: Ingegerd and I arrived in Arlington, Va. visited Mt. Vernon
Aug. 24: Drove from Arlington to Croton-on-Hudson, N.Y.

Just after Ingegerd left for Sweden September 10 on the Gripsholm, Signe picked up her normal work schedule. It was back to Metropolitan Life Insurance and more time spent on the amputee manual.

To practice physical therapy in New York State, one had to be licensed by examination or by endorsement. According to information obtained from the New York State Education

Department, Signe was licensed under the "grandfather" clause and special provisions of statute on June 3, 1953. Her ID number was "613A", and Dr. Kristieng Hansson, of the Hospital for Special Surgery, was listed as her supervisor.

On September 2, 1953, the day after having a conference with Dr. Donald Covalt, Signe started to work at New York University—in Bellevue Medical Center's Institute for Physical Medicine and Rehabilitation, in the Prosthetic Department. She also maintained a role as a consultant with the Kessler Institute. In what spare time she had, Signe diligently worked to complete the amputee manual. She went to Lodi to meet with Don Kerr but the surroundings provided "interferences all day." This proved very frustrating for Signe, who preferred to work quietly and alone at Bullet Hole. It was not until February 11, 1954, that the manuscript *Training the Lower Extremity Amputee* was sent to Charles C Thomas, Publisher, in Springfield, Illinois. That was not the end of the project. There still would be a great deal of work to be done.

Francoise Lamote met Signe again at the Institute of Physical Medicine and Rehabilitation in 1954. In a recent letter, she described an interesting anecdote:

> I worked at the Institute where I found Signe was a P.T. consultant. I knew Donald Kerr and I admired the work they did together at the Kessler Institute. One day, Signe invited me and a friend to her home on Bullet Hole Road to spend a weekend and relax. It was the most amazing relaxing weekend I ever spent in my life. At 6 A.M., I woke up and found Signe cutting wood for the barbecue. I could only do one thing—go and help her. At breakfast, she started explaining her research on hemiplegia. It was so interesting we didn't see the time lost. The whole weekend was PT research, hemiplegia, work, PT again. I went back to work on Monday morning completely exhausted and tired after a wonderful "relaxing weekend." Signe didn't even realize how much we worked during the weekend! She came back to the Institute and said to me, "You seem

to be interested in my work on hemiplegia, so I'll come after work to show you my patient, and show you the results.'' And she did it!

When Signe finished her book on hemiplegia, she sent me a copy with the following inscription:

''To Francoise, With admiration for your outstanding achievements and your devotion to rehabilitation; and in remembrance of our personal friendship.''

Francoise's comments about Signe continued. She wrote:

> Since 1954, I have always been using Signe's methods and always had outstanding achievement. I taught her method to my students and I am about to write a paper for the local therapists. I think she was the best PT I ever met and the most enthusiastic and intense person I knew. She lived PT, worked PT, slept PT. She was a brain and I loved her. But it was very difficult to keep up with her. She was too intense, too strong. Nobody could follow her. She extenuated anybody who tried. She was a ''plus'' but too hard to follow.

On March 8, 1954, Signe made a telephone call to Tony DeRosa, Chief of the Physical Therapy Department at the Burke Foundation Rehabilitation Center in White Plains, New York. She requested a visit and wished to discuss extending her research with hemiplegic patients. Dr. Edward Lorenze was medical director at Burke when Signe joined the staff. He was very supportive of her research, and according to Tony DeRosa, would often repeat: ''I would love to discover the answer to the functional rehabilitation of the hemiplegic upper extremity.'' Tony described what followed:

> Here I was a 1949 graduate from N.Y.U., having practiced at the Institute for Rehabilitation Medicine for two years and then accepting an appointment at Burke to assist in developing a comprehensive rehabilitation program . . . indeed a neophyte therapist working hard to advance physical therapy care . . . and Signe Brunnstrom of whom I have heard and read so much, who represented one of the moving forces in our

> clinical world wanted to "work" with us. Dr. Lorenze was delighted, staff was in awe and I was "speechless," but we forged ahead. Nothing was more surprising to us at the Burke P.T. department, than the arrival of Signe, ready to work! Not withstanding the notoriety Signe enjoyed throughout the physical therapy world-community, she came to Burke very quietly, unassuming, modest and almost "walking on her toes" lest she in any way "offend" the regular staff members—be they therapists, nurses or physicians. I thought "if only she realized how much we looked forward to her working with us and sharing her wealth of knowledge."
>
> Signe's power of observation, her knowledge of kinesiology, anatomy and neurology, and her feelings for the disabled, were truly beautiful to behold as one observed her evaluation and treatment of patients.

Signe gave unstintingly of herself. Tony observed that she always had time to answer a question from a staff member or a student. "Signe radiated," Tony recalled, "and her smile was soothing and put one at ease, as she proceeded to explain a response."

Tony also felt that much of accepted treatment of neurologically-impaired patients needed something more dynamic. "It appeared that we were at a stand still-range of motion, some attempts at therapeutic exercise (which did not bring forth significant volitional movements) and ADL training. There was a need for more." According to Tony, "Signe provided that innovative and dynamic approach. Her associated motions, her mass muscle movements, her heavy reliance on neurophysiology, has truly opened a new dimension to the management of the hemiplegic patient." Commenting on the value of Signe's work, Tony stated, "I am convinced that her approach has thus far stood the test of time. It is still the best approach from the standpoint of basis in neurophysiology and results achieved." He has hopes that other physical therapists will continue to add to the research Signe has so well initiated. To this end, it became obvious that all of the material and observations Signe noted had to be compiled. Tony recalls sitting for hours with Signe discussing how this could be done. Signe decided to prepare rough drafts of the material, which became the "manual", outlining in a progressive manner her approach to treating the hemiplegic patient. The material was the forerunner of Signe's third major publication. In those early days at Burke, Tony DeRosa played a very important role in assisting Signe with the manual. He was responsible for scheduling of patients; obtaining necessary consent forms; providing for facilities; and arranging for the first mimeograph printing of the manual in the Burke Vocational Rehabilitation Services printing shop. "I recall 26 copies were printed for the exclusive use of Signe's students at Columbia," Tony related recently. Signe was very concerned that the copies be limited, as she knew that someday in the future, the material could be the basis of a publication. (Eventually, according to Signe's notes, 150 copies were made of the manual.)

In the Spring of 1954, Signe decided to list her Hill House for sale. She received three offers through real estate people, but took no immediate action. It was apparent that she could obtain an income by renting the upstairs and the downstairs as two apartments. By mid-May, she had the upper level rented to a Mr. and Mrs. Hoffman, only to be disappointed when they canceled the rental a few days later. But she was able to rent the entire house for July and August to "Mr. and Mrs. Donnelly and young child," as her diary states.

At one point during her work at the Burke Foundation, Signe told Tony DeRosa her house needed some repairs. Tony relates the story that Signe actually asked for "a few days off while she did the repairs. She was indeed a most unusual person that one would not easily forget."

Again, in September, she placed Hill House up for sale. Living in the renovated "coop" suited Signe's needs. The very term "chicken coop" conjures in one's mind a place less than habitable for a human being, but this coop was different. What Signe did with the wooden shack demonstrated another of her unique traits—simplicity. Martha Schnebly, and Ruth Dickinson, teaching assistants at Columbia, both visited Signe in Putnam County. Martha offered a description of what she found:

> Signe had a house, barn and chicken coop on a few acres of land, but what she had done was convert the chicken house into her home and rented the main house. That chicken house made a most attractive home and it seemed to suit her to a T. It contained four rooms in a row, the living room took the full width at one end, then a hallway lead past the kitchen and bath and into the bedroom that filled the opposite end of the house. A row of small windows ran along the high side of house under the roof's edge which gave a lovely indirect light into the rooms and hallway. It was a plain structure but reflected the warmth and simplicity of her Swedish background.

"It was a charming country home," according to Ruth Dickinson, "one that Signe personally made over from an 'honest-to-goodness chicken coop'. The inside decor was simple, uncluttered 'modern Swedish', with soft muted colors and hand woven pillow cases and coverlettes. The outside area was natural, rocky, full of trees and hilly." Every year Signe would clear away the underbrush and expand the grassy area. How did Signe accomplish all of the work? Sometimes she had help, as described by Ruth who visited Bullet Hole Road on many occasions while still working at the Kessler Institute:

> In those early 1950's our P.T. staff had some wonderful social times with Signe. During visits to Carmel, she always put us to work and we practically thanked her for that. The several big burly men on our staff, the spouse of one of our women members along with Signe moved the boulders and cut and carted the wood. We lesser folk trimmed the forsythia from around the barn. It was really funny. Signe and the men doing all the heavy stuff and we other women doing the lighter chores!

Signe had a special friendly relationship with Fran Tappan, Director of the Physical Therapy program at the The University of Connecticut in Storrs. The university was one of Signe's favorite educational facilities. Signe and Fran Tappan were close friends for many years. Their friendship went back to a meeting at Stanford University when Fran was studying under Margaret Rood. Occasionally Signe and Don Kerr traveled to Storrs to give a lecture on amputees. Following Signe's talk, Don gave a demonstration of how well an amputee could function. At other times, Signe lectured to the senior physical therapy students on muscle testing of the shoulder girdle, biomechanics of standing and locomotion, the physiological basis for Kabat-Kaiser, muscle action, and peripheral nerve injuries.

Fran often related a story about Signe and her determination. On September 11, 1954, at Fran's invitation, Signe drove to Storrs to present a lecture on "Associated Reactions in Hemiplegia," as part of a large educational conference. That was the weekend of "Hurricane Carol". Parts of the New England coast and Long Island were devastated. Signe was determined to get to the university, and she did! She arrived at Fran's house and there was no electrical power. The conference was canceled. Rather than seek accommodations at a nearby motel, Signe encouraged a handful of faculty to stick it out. Supper was cooked over a fireplace, and Signe decided to use the time for a lecture-review. By candlelight, the small group listened intently as she discussed various techniques such as Rood and Knott. She recommended that every therapist take the best of everything and make sense out of it. Signe felt there was something good in every approach and it would be wrong to settle just for one way of treating a patient. (Actually Signe did not approve of the term "Brunnstrom Approach." She felt all approaches had some similarities, and at times one could not tell whose name should be associated with a certain technique.)

The group worked throughout the night of the hurricane and Signe went home the next day. In talking about Signe, Fran stated, "I am glad she was published. Once you publish you become immortal. Signe's personality is a legacy in itself. She had strength of character. She could get angry, but was one of the most pleasant persons I have ever known." Fran Tappan, a legend in her own right, may be counted among the many physical therapists who were greatly influenced by Signe.

As 1954 came to an end, Signe and Don Kerr were still working on revisions of the amputee manual. While the publisher had accepted the manuscript, many changes had to be made. Signe had asked T. Campbell Thompson, M.D., of the Hospital for Special Surgery, to review the manuscript and write the introduction. He agreed. His final paragraph stated:

> The reader of this manual is indeed fortunate to have the experience of these two authors combined in one volume. It is with great pleasure that I recommend it to all amputees, and to all others who are interested in amputee rehabilitation.

By April 25, 1955, the galley proofs for the amputee manual arrived at Signe's home. The well-illustrated 272 page hard cover book was actually published by Charles C Thomas, and made available early in 1956. Its preparation was a major part of Signe's life for almost six years! In an attempt to obtain a copy of the original contract and to find out how many books were published and sold, I corresponded with Payne Thomas. He replied: "I wish that we could cooperate with you in furnishing the information which you have requested. It has always been our policy, however, not to furnish information on sales to anyone except the author. Similarly, it has always been our policy not to furnish copies of agreements to anyone except the author. We trust you will understand our position." Don Kerr related a story about the number of books sold. He was aware that sales were 50 short of the number needed to require the publisher to pay royalties. He suggested to Signe that he and she split the purchase of the books. This would then result in their being paid some royalties. Signe did not appreciate the idea, and according to Don, "just didn't understand what I was trying to do."

Throughout 1955, Signe worked at several positions. She was involved with the Burke Rehab Center, teaching at Columbia, and consulting at NYU-IRM. She continued lecturing at physical therapy meetings and in various hospitals, worked on a film, prepared some manuscripts and treated private patients.

At the Burke Center, during a lull in the research program, Signe asked Tony DeRosa "for permission" to work with an amputee patient. "It was a delightful experience," Tony reported, "to observe her manner and clinical approach. Her interest was centered on the neurologic approach to hemiplegia, but she never lost the feel for the value of physical therapy for all disabilities."

With her teaching at Columbia, Signe expressed some "apprehension and concern" over her course in Kinesiology. In conversations with Tony DeRosa, she expressed her fear that her knowledge and practical experience would overwhelm the students, and that they would not gain sufficiently from her teachings. Tony felt that time proved her fears and apprehensions were merely an expression of her depth of interest on behalf of the students who "truly loved their teacher."

On June 26, 1955, Signe went to Rock Hill, Connecticut and renewed her acquaintance with Herb Jones. He recalled the situation:

> We were able to get Signe to come to the hospital for a demonstration and lecture on her work and treatment techniques for hemiplegics which greatly influenced our treatment program. It just happened that the Connecticut Chapter of the APTA (I was Program Chairman at the time) wanted to have her talk. The chapter was small and poor in the purse in those days. Signe realized that and said in place of her usual honorarium, she would be glad to have the train fare to Manchester where she was going to be the next day. We were overjoyed and as Manchester is only twenty miles from Rocky Hill, I told the chapter officers that it wouldn't cost us a cent since I would drive her to Manchester

after the meeting. WELL!, the morning she arrived at the hospital, she gave me her schedule for the day and evening and asked if in the evening she could speak first and the chapter have the business meeting later after she left. She said she had checked with the railroad and the train left about 11PM. I told Signe 'No need for a train, I'll drive you.' Signe said, "All the way to Manchester, New Hampshire?" I blanched—we all thought she meant our local Manchester. Needless to say we scurried around getting contributions to pay for the train ticket.

Years later I met her at a dinner meeting and spoke about the experience. She said she never realized it and we all had a good laugh. I was always impressed by Signe's ability to go into an area with full immersion, learning all about it and then working with hands on—directly with the patient, writing for journals and texts and then on to another area of the field. Very few can match her versatility. Signe influenced me to become proficient in a few areas so I have concentrated in prosthetic-orthotic training and geriatrics. The profession owes a lot to her.

In 1956, Jack Hofkosh, aware of Signe's work with the amputees at IRM, spoke with Doctors Rusk, Covalt and Lowman on Signe's behalf, to assist in arranging for a part-time research and clinical activity program in the physical therapy department. According to Jack, "Here is where Signe demonstrated some of her first clinical trials of developing research into the 'associated motion patterns.' We all learned much from Signe; her patience, her tolerance and her professional acumen endeared this wonderful woman to all of us privileged to have worked with her during the years 1956 through 1961."

Gerald Stern of Baldwin, New York is Chief Physical Therapist at The Community Hospital at Glen Cove in Glen Cove, New York. He was a staff physical therapist at IRM in 1956–57. At that time the physical therapy department was reorganizing its treatment program procedures into disability groups. In a letter of August 9, 1987, Gerald described the situation:

> Signe, myself and two other therapists were assigned to treat all of the C.V.A.'s. Signe was the leader of our treatment team and she trained us in her techniques which we utilized for muscle reeducation reinforcment procedures as well as gait training. She was both knowledgeable and dynamic and was able to elicit movements from paralyzed extremities that not only awed her peers but left the medical staff almost inadequate in comprehending the necessary blending of both her scientific rationale and artistic techniques. All of her patients loved her. All of the therapists respected her abilities but her pioneering in neuromuscular facilitation techniques combined with her dogmatic personality, caused some friction with the medical staff and eventually, I believe, contributed to her departure from the Institute. I personally found Signe to be a delight to work with and the facilitation techniques that she taught me served to make me a much better therapist and I am sure contributed greatly to the success of my career. I often think of her and I will always be thankful for the privilege of knowing and working with this GREAT WOMAN.

Virginia Consiglio met Signe Brunnstrom at the Institute for Rehab Medicine in 1956. Recalling her acquaintance with Signe she stated (in a letter of December 13, 1984), "I was fortunate to receive her teachings through the patients who attended the out-patient clinics." Virginia exercised her physical therapy skills in Buenos Aires for 20 years (from 1957 through 1977). She felt the education received under Signe gave her many advantages when working in Argentina:

> The polio epidemic that broke out in 1955 and 1956 in my country demanded the assistance of many sources from abroad, expertise as well as equipment, to undertake the organization of specialized services for the numerous victims of the disease. An Association to

> Fight Against Polio (ALPI) created through the efforts of the parents of the stricken youngsters, launched a country-wide campaign to provide rehabilitation services.
>
> The Institute Marcelo J. Fitts, under the auspices of ALPI became the center for services. It was there that I became intensively engaged in the field of physical therapy. As the scope of the services expanded, the care of the adult hemiplegic became obvious. I had the opportunity to apply the teachings of Miss Brunnstrom and to demonstrate a technique far different from the Sister Kenny method. The idea of using links of movements through the ''flexion and extension'' synergies of the limbs and its relation to that of the head and trunk, disclosed a new approach in the treatment of the upper motor neuron lesion which enhanced the motor responses and function of these patients. The prolific bibliography and works of numerous researchers in the field of neurophysiology so uniquely compiled by Signe became enlightening reading material for the practitioner.

Virginia also wrote, ''It was around 1965 that I contacted Signe with reference to having her book translated into Spanish. After getting in touch with the publisher under her suggestion, a number of inconveniences besides economical adversities unfortunately precluded the concretion of this project.'' (Actually, the first edition of the book in Spanish was published in 1977, with a second printing in 1979. The Spanish version, *Reeducacion Motora En La Hemiplejia—Fundamentos Neurofisiologicos,* was prepared by Maria Victoria Carbo De Valls and published by Editorial JIMS, Barcelona 6, Spain.)

The Second World Confederation for Physical Therapy, Second Congress was held in New York June 17–23, 1956. On Tuesday, June 19, Signe was part of an afternoon session in which she presented a half-hour lecture on ''The Use of Associated Reaction Patterns in the Training of Adult Patients with Hemiplegia.''

Anyone who has ever written a professional article is aware of the amount of time it takes. How Signe found time in 1955 and 1956 to write three major articles in between her other responsibilities further demonstrates the dedication she had to the profession. The articles were *Methods to Elicit, Reinforce and Coordinate Muscular Response in Upper Motor Lesions in the APTA-OVR Institute Papers,* (1956); *The use of associated reactions patterns in the training of adult patients with hemiplegia in the proceedings of the Second Congress, World Confederation for Physical Therapy,* (1956); and *Associated Reactions of the Upper Extremity in Adult Patients with Hemiplegia, An Approach to Training,* in the (Physical Therapy Review, 1956).

Paul J. Collura, DDS, lived on Bullet Hole Road almost seven years before he and his wife really got to know Signe since she did not bother much with her neighbors. "Her external demeanor was severe," he wrote on March 11, 1986, "her countenance, stern. Her lined face and deep set dark eyes accentuated this severity. In essence though, she was a gentle, understanding and compassionate person." He also recalled that Signe was "up with the break of first light and could work through the whole day." Dr. Collura was amazed at how she tackled boulders and moved them, cleared the land and then landscaped it. As a neighbor, he did not particularly like her dogs. He saw them as being "protective and possessive of her," and she in return maintained a very similar attitude towards them. To describe the true essence of Signe, Dr. Collura related a special incident that occurred in 1957:

> In July my home was struck by lightning and burned to the ground. I left the Carmel area for about two months after this fire. I found temporary living quarters some thirty miles from Carmel. During this time of commuting between office and temporary home, I was made aware of the fact that Signe was looking for me. I called on her. Compassionately, she showed concern for my family and inquired what my plans were for a future home. She was aware that my children

went to school in Carmel and that they would be hard-pressed what with the tragedy of the fire and now the possibility of changing schools if we remained away from Carmel. She offered me the Hill House totally furnished! I was deeply moved and and impressed, but felt I couldn't accept her offer because I didn't want to see her go back to living in the converted coop. She explained that living in the coop wasn't necessary because with a few alterations she could make an apartment for herself in the garage below the Hill House. On this condition, I accepted her offer and spoke to her about financial arrangements. She made the offer totally free of charge. I wouldn't accept that and finally we worked out something suitable but at a minimum cost because she wouldn't have it any other way.

Referring to Signe's struggle with the state and the highway construction, Dr. Collura indicated that Signe "lived in terror of the State." He stated, "She felt to fight was futile because they held condemnation of the property as a penalty over her head. The thought of having her beloved acreage and orchard destroyed, depressed her terribly." Signe also became Dr. Collura's patient for many years.

As an instructor in the programs for physical and occupational therapy students at the College of Physicians and Surgeons at Columbia University, Signe influenced many therapists and left them with lasting impressions. One such person was George P. Jessup, Jr. (now living in Panama City, Florida). He wrote:

During the period of time in which I was on the faculty at Columbia University I served as the teaching assistant and kinesiological model for Signe Brunnstrom. There were certain of the student body who did not appreciate having a live individual demonstrating muscle functioning, sometimes somewhat semi-nude. Later on when Signe wrote her textbook on kinesiology as you know she used extensive stick figures. I always felt that she was able to draw those figures from memory of what she had me performing before the classes. Another individual who worked at the College of Physicians and Surgeons at Columbia, as a teaching assistant to Signe, was an occupational therapist named Martha Schnebly. She wrote:

> There are a number of words that come to mind when I think of Signe—vigor, intensity, singleness of purpose, orderly minded, warm and gentle spirit, quiet sense of humor, sensitivity. She is one of those rare people whose beauty of spirit shines through her rather plain exterior.

Referring to Signe as a teacher, Martha continues,

> In the classroom she made every effort to help students learn. She wanted every student to be successful in understanding the principles and application of kinesiology. She would explain, demonstrate and question to make her concepts and knowledge clear and she could laugh when her accent led to some misunderstandings. She was always actively learning while teaching.

Between 1957 and 1959, Signe collaborated with Dr. Glenn Reynolds of the Institute of Physical Medicine and Rehabilitation in co-authoring three major articles. The first was an unpublished, mimeographed Report on the Study of Neurophysiological Reactions Facilitating Recovery Following Hemiplegia. This was followed by a published article in the Archives of Physical Medicine and Rehabilitation, (Vol. 39:303, 1958), *Preliminary Report on Neuromuscular Function Testing of the Upper Extremity in Adult Hemiplegia Patients*. In 1959, Rehabilitation Literature, (Vol. 20:163), carried their article, *Problems of Sensorimotor Learning in the Evaluation and Treatment of the Adult Hemiplegic Patient*. Dr. Reynolds also worked with Signe on two films, "Training of the Arm in Adult Patients with Hemiplegia," and "Neurophysiologic Influences in the Restoration of Function in Adult Patients with Hemiplegia." The films were available from NYU's Film Library.

While teaching Kinesiology at Columbia in the spring of 1959, Signe saw the need for a special manual to assist the students in their study of kinesiology. With the support and encouragement of Mary Callahan, director of the physical therapy program, Ruth Dickinson, Assistant Director, and Dr. Robert Darling, Medical Director, she developed a teaching grant application for the preparation of a kinesiology laboratory manual. (This was not the manual developed at the Burke Rehabilitation facility.) The application was submitted to the Office of Vocational Rehabilitation and the actual grant was approved on August 22, 1959. Preparation of the publication would take several years, and one can wonder if Signe ever realized what a major contribution the text would be to students and personnel in the field of rehabilitation.

With the knowledge that the grant was confirmed, Signe accepted an invitation to give a workshop on hemiplegia in Daytona Beach, at the meeting of the Florida Chapter of APTA October 9–10. The late Fred Rutan, (passed away November 23, 1988) of Albuquerque, a recently-graduated physical therapist at that time, attended the conference. He recalled the meeting (in a letter of January 2, 1985) as his first continuing education program after graduation:

> Even though I went to New York University, I never met Signe until I got to Florida. It was quite a learning experience for a new physical therapist. I was very impressed with the fact that here was a name Elizabeth Addoms had mentioned through school and I was finally able to take a course with her.

Another physical therapist at the Daytona workshop was Sue Hirt. She offered an interesting insight into Signe's character:

> I remember at the workshop, Signe and I were wading barefoot on the beach in the dark thoroughly enjoying the experience and each other. Signe was a rather reserved and very intense person. It was not easy to come to know her, but when I had the chance to spend a few moments alone with her, I felt the warmth, ma-

> turity, and above all, the incredible strength of conviction that her role in life was to improve the existence of the handicapped. It was almost overwhelming. I believe Signe has opened our eyes for seeing and seeking the scientific basis for understanding the clinical picture and appropriate treatment procedures. When you watched her treating a patient you had the feeling that she slipped inside the patient's skin and could feel what it was like to struggle for return to normal living.

After the Florida meeting, Signe attended the conference of the American Occupational Therapy Association (AOTA) in Chicago, and on return to Putnam County, she moved out of the cottage to her larger Hill House. This gave her more room to work on the kinesiology manuscript. However, she had an opportunity to rent the house, and since she could use the funds, it was back to the cottage. Every spare moment was devoted to the manuscript.

The final manual that led to the text *Clinical Kinesiology* will be a living tribute to Signe as it continues to be one of the most important publications available to physical and occupational therapy students. Developing the actual manuscript and finalizing the galleys for publication took three years. All of the manuscript preparation and typing, page by page, was done on her own time. Signe could not afford to just sit home and write. Added to her work responsibilities was: serving as a consultant to the Veterans Administration Regional Office; traveling to Walter Reed Hospital in Washington; flying to Indianapolis and to Richmond to give lectures; preparing an article on motor behavior for the *Journal of Occupational Therapy*; and organizing a two-week course for the New York State Rehabilitation Hospital at West Haverstraw.

On June 1, 1961, Signe signed a contract with the F.A. Davis Publishing Company for publication of *Clinical Kinesiology*. The contract, signed by, Frank Craven President, stated that: "(the) AUTHOR agrees to deliver the completed manuscript for said book to PUBLISHER, within eighteen months from this date of agreement . . . " For her work,

Signe was to receive 10 percent of the net wholesale price at which the book was sold, (The net wholesale price being understood to be 25 percent less than the retail price on all copies sold). The price of the book was $6.50. Signe received about 48 cents per book sold in this country. For export copies, the royalty was 50 percent of the usual royalty—or 24 cents—because of the lower prices received from foreign sales. The eventual income from the book would be in the thousands of dollars, but Signe in her own altruistic way would not see the full benefit. (More on that later.)

As part of the preparation of the new text, Signe needed photographs. Ruth Dickinson recalled the events that led to finding the right model:

> Signe wanted to include photos of a person with 'normal' musculature and she had negotiated with a local photographer to take pictures. She needed to find a suitable subject who could be easily available. Althea Jones of the Columbia faculty had a friend who directed a summer camp near Carmel and we hit on the thought that perhaps a camp counselor (young, healthy, muscular) could be found to pose. So we, with Signe, visited the camp and she made her selection and the young man agreed to help.

Signe must have appreciated the time and effort expended by the "model", as she recognized his contribution in the book's acknowledgment: "The author also wishes to extend her thanks to the young man who patiently served as a model for a great many photographs in this book."

Before getting deeply involved in finalizing the manuscript, she left on Loftleider (Icelandic) Airlines July 31 for a six-week visit to Sweden.

Upon returning August 28, Signe was back to the busy schedule which included teaching Kinesiology 105 and Kinesiology 206 at Columbia, serving as a consultant at the VA, conducting an OT study course at the Neurological Institute, seeing private patients and preparing the new manuscript. In her notes, Signe emphasized the amount of work that went into the project, " . . . 1962 typed Clinical Kinesiology book manuscript."

Martha Schnebly, OTR, was very familiar with Signe's concern for producing a perfect text.

> Signe wrote her textbook during the years Ruth Dickinson and I assisted her. Her first effort was a typed manual with photographs which we used in class for at least one year before she would allow it to go to the publishers. She took such care in its preparation that at times we doubted if it would ever be written to her satisfaction. In spite of some of its early shortcomings, she gave our "fields of work" a book unique to our practices at a time when we had little to go on except what physical educators published. She made us focus on palpation and daily functions, rather than athletics.

On April 27, 1962, a corrected manuscript was mailed to the publisher. Two months later, on June 12, Signe traveled to Philadelphia to meet with the publishers, and a month later, she had the first galleys. In the preface to the first edition of the text, published in 1962, Signe indicated that she used the contents of the book for years in teaching kinesiology to physical and occupational therapy students:

> The original manual was then revised and enlarged to include material on certain aspects of pathological motor behavior. The clinical aspects of kinesiology were given emphasis to meet the needs of workers in the field of rehabilitation of the physically handicapped.

In recent correspondence (January 4, 1984) commenting on the success of the publication, Robert H. Craven, President of F.A. Davis wrote:

> This has been a worthwhile book in many ways. It has been a great success for the F.A. Davis Company, it has been practically a necessity for every student and

> you may be interested to know it has been one of our best selling books in Europe.

Signe would gain international fame as a result of the published text. *Clinical Kinesiology,* her second book, would prove to be quite demanding of her time, so much so that, in years to come, she would relinquish the rights to the third edition to her dear friend, Ruth Dickinson.

Despite the effort and energy expenditure required to see the text come to fruition, Signe was not through with writing. It was not the royalties or the recognition she wanted. Her commitment was to share knowledge with other professionals. At a time in life when many people consider retiring, Signe, at age 64, was involved in a most time-consuming project, and she knew the work must be done! The text has stood the test of time, with the third edition revised by Dickinson in 1972, and a fourth edition by Don Lehmkuhl and Laura Smith in 1983, who are also preparing the fifth edition. Even with the amount of work the text required, Signe already conceived the idea of preparing another major publication based on the manual mimeographed at the Burke Foundation dealing with therapy for the hemiplegic. (More on this in a later connection.)

Signe's teaching at Columbia had a profound effect on many people. Mary Callahan, former director of the physical therapy program, recalled the relationship she had with Signe:

> I can see her now, bursting into the school office, exuding quantities of energy, flushed in the face and eager to discuss her teaching, the students or the books being developed. I dropped whatever I was doing, tried to present a relaxed manner, as at times I felt her blood pressure was "sky high!" In retrospect I believe she would have felt better had I become intense too! I am proud of the books developed under government grants in spite of many frustrations. Signe was a perfectionist of the highest order. She belonged to the school "where you did everything yourself." Delegation of responsibilities for the grant was not in her nature. We

> even had to reconcile our differences with the financial office. However, we made it together, had many laughs and good times.
>
> I am also proud of the quality of her teaching. She was dedicated and expected every student to absorb material. A final grade of less that a B+ distressed her! All students should be in the A range.

One would think that with the first edition of *Clinical Kinesiology* now published, Signe would have taken a vacation. That was not the case. On February 23, 1963, she started writing an article on gait analysis in hemiplegia. It was completed and mailed on October 3 to Helen Hislop, then editor of the Journal of Physical Therapy. (The article was published in Vol. 44 No. 1: pages 11–14,1964.)

In March, April and May, Signe continued teaching kinesiology 105 and 206 at Columbia. She lectured on hand rehabilitation at Grace New Haven Hospital on April 6; conducted a training program on evaluation of the adult patient with hemiplegia in St. Paul, Minnesota on May 9; and attended the APTA Conference in New York City on May 29. In one of the sessions she heard a lecture on hand research given by Mary Eleanor Brown and Lorraine Lake. Mary Eleanor recollected:

> I hadn't seen Signe for 15 years and I remember how flattered I was to see her in my audience at another national conference. I was presenting the Cleveland Hand Research being conducted at Highland View Hospital. When I was making the electrodes it was natural for me to insert them into my own hands and forearms. I often thought of watching Signe relating every step of her inquiries to her own muscles. Many of my most successful visual aids were made from my own x-rays, electromyograms and electrogoniograms. Signe was an applied kinesiologist of the highest order.

During the spring of 1963, Signe also was involved in one of her first loves, that of making films. Working with Samuel Feitelberg at the Neurological Institute, at New York's

Columbia-Presbyterian Medical Center, various patients were photographed. Sam, presently serving as Professor and Chairperson of the Department of Physical Therapy at the University of Vermont, recalled the experience in a letter of November 13, 1985:

> We made a film of her techniques, and I had the good fortune to operate the camera. She knew exactly what she wanted to accomplish. Every moment was a learning experience. Her respect for the patient was a sight to behold. What she made them feel was evidenced by what they did for her. I have seen few patients work as hard for their therapist.
>
> She started her day with energy and the feeling of "let's go to work," wasting no time and being prepared. She always ended with a smile and a feeling of accomplishment and exhaustion. Her name Signe, must be appropriate . . . a signal or sign to follow. Her patients did just that for her and for themselves. Her students could never get enough of her light.

On June 22, Signe received a teaching offer from Stanford University to teach kinesiology since Marian Williams, the instructor, became ill. Signe accepted the offer and contacted her older sister, Elsa, in Sweden. The plan was for Elsa to visit this country and drive with Signe to California. Elsa arrived at Bullet Hole on October 22. On November 6, with two dogs in the car, they set off for a cross-country trip. (This was the second such drive for Signe the first was in 1953.) Once again, Signe kept a detailed account of the trip, describing the scenery, accommodations, roads, crops, and special sights.

Bypassing Durham, North Carolina, Signe decided to stop at Chapel Hill, at the University of North Carolina to visit a well-known physical therapist and educator, Margaret L. Moore. Margaret (now retired in Holly Ridge, North Carolina) recalls the visit:

> I didn't know Signe personally—only admired her from afar—for the thoroughness of her work, her ded-

ication to patients and her enthusiasm. She did come to Chapel Hill in 1963, but unannounced! She just walked in the door and it took a while for secretaries and staff to come and find me. She was just going through town.

On the 11th, Signe and Elsa visited the Georgia Warm Springs Foundation. While there, Signe gave a demonstration on two hemiplegic patients before the PT and OT staff and 15 foreign trainees. This was followed by a "cocktail party at Kathryn Phillip's place."

The next several days were spent driving across Alabama, part of Mississippi, Louisiana and into Texas. When they got to the Carlsbad Caverns, Signe felt it was too hot to leave the dogs in the car, so she placed them in a kennel. The caverns trip involved an hour-and-a-quarter hike on trails and 700 feet down an elevator, although Signe was 65 and Elsa 68! Signe's notes indicate, "From Carlsbad we did not drive to El Paso (too hot), instead north to Artesia, overnight in Cloudcraft in Lincoln National Forest, altitude 8,640 feet."

The drive continued "over a dry Rio Grande at San Antonio," north via Pueblo to an Indian reservation, after passing Albuquerque. Due to "heavy rain and snow in the mountains," Signe and Elsa stopped at Cuba, New Mexico on Route 44. The next morning the car was "iced over" due to the rain and frost, but Signe decided to move on to Farmington, New Mexico, to visit an old friend, Elfriede Prins.

Elfriede (then Werthmann) first met Signe in 1932 in New York City when she was a student in the physical therapy course at the Hospital for Ruptured and Crippled. She wrote about Signe (October 4, 1986); "What I mostly remember about Signe is her friendship. I was alone in the city as a teen-ager, with no friends and no relatives. I too, as an immigrant, found a friend in Signe, and an inspiration to excel in my work. I learned from her what no college could have provided, the motivation to excel."

"One Christmas," Elfriede recalled, "Signe gave us a party, second to none, at her top floor apartment in the city. She had a Christmas tree with candles, lute fish, and all trimmings, grog too. About five of us slept on the floor. Signe told me a Swedish friend gave all the refreshments and he didn't want anybody to know who he was. We all, except Signe, were poor. Today I thought about it for the first time, maybe Signe provided all the goodies!''

After completing the course, Elfriede moved to Seattle. Signe visited with her during the Navy years in Mare Island. Later, in 1958, Elfriede and her 12-year-old son Richard, stayed with Signe at her Putnam County home. Signe, apparently was very fond of Richard. During their brief stay, only one problem arose, one of Signe's dog's bit Richard. He remembers that to this day!

As to the visit by Signe and Elsa on November 17 and 18, 1963, Elfriede recalled having several friends, including two Indians, as dinner guests to meet her visitors from New York and Sweden. One of the Indians was Tecumseh, an Oklahoman and an x-ray technician at the local hospital. His recollection of Signe included her owning ''two well trained, well mannered dogs.''

Another dinner guest, Christine Durham, also recalled the dinner. Referring to Signe, she wrote, ''I remember her quite well. She was very gracious and made it very easy for me to talk to her about Texas and the cotton industry.'' Alice Jackson, a Navajo, was also a dinner guest.

Elfriede remembered that Signe once mentioned she had Elk meat in Sweden for Christmas, so she decided to make Elk for dinner. The meat was given to her by a former patient and she had saved it for a special occasion. Both Signe and Elsa enjoyed the dinner and the company very much. ''I can see her now,'' wrote Elfriede, ''sitting in my kitchen. During dinner I was busy serving and noticed Signe and Tecumseh talking. I helped more with Elsa and Mrs. Durham because Elsa knew better German than English. Mr. Durham told Elsa how the cotton grows in Texas and all about the squash we brought back from the Bolack's Agricultural Research and Experimental Farm.''

Later, Signe and Elfriede talked about the old times in New York. They discussed the physician who called Signe ''a traitor to medicine'' because she wouldn't agree to be called a "technician". Years later, that physician changed his mind about Signe when he read her articles on treatment for the CVA patient.

The next day, Signe and Elsa visited the local hospital with Elfriede. They also saw the experimental farm and some Aztec ruins. That was the last time Elfriede saw Signe.

On December 9, 1986, Elfriede, wrote:

> I am sad to hear about her condition now. The best compliment I ever had in my life was when someone called me "Little Miss Brunnstrom." I am almost 80 years old now, but all this memory brings tears to my eyes, all of us pioneers have a lot to be thankful for to Signe—and I most of all.

Signe and Elsa left Farmington on November 20 and headed to Tuba City, Cameron and the Grand Canyon. At the Canyon, they hit a snowstorm but went on to Prescott. By November 22, they were over the Weaver Mountains and into the cactus area. Signe notes they drove through "100 miles of desert with mountain views, then citrus groves, vineyards all the way to Los Angeles."

It was while driving through L.A. to Woodland Hills on November 23 that they heard the shocking news of President Kennedy's assassination. "This explained all the flags on half-mast we had seen when driving that day," she wrote. That evening they arrived at Carmel-on-the-Sea. Sunday morning, they attended mass at Carmel Mission for President Kennedy. The evening was spent with a former Navy colleague, Shirley Mainwaring. Lucille Daniels met Signe on November 25 for a conference about the teaching schedule and course. Thanksgiving was spent with Shirley and Thomas Mainwaring. Signe then found a cottage to share with Peggy McGivert during the teaching assignment.

The night before Elsa had to head East, they had dinner with Lucille Daniels. The next morning, Elsa boarded the Zephyr and headed for Chicago to catch the 20th Century Limited. Once in New York, she took a Scandinavian Air Lines flight for home.

In California, Signe reviewed her material, read Mary Fiorentino's book on reflex testing methods and spent a week preparing for Kinesiology 220. Thanks to the kindness of Sarah Semans, Signe was not alone on Christmas, 1963. Sarah invited her for Christmas dinner. Present also were Sarah's father and some other invited guests. Sarah recalled that afternoon in a letter December 12, 1984 from Palo Alto:

> I knew Signe personally only briefly. That was when she was at Stanford taking over Marian William's teaching program during Marian's illness. It was at that time that Signe had Christmas dinner with us in Menlo Park. But Signe had a great influence on me professionally. What I remember first was Marian's account of Signe's studies on muscle function of the shoulder, done, I believe while in the Navy. Then when I was teaching Kinesiology, I used her text book as the best then available. Her work with stroke patients fascinated me, as I watched her demonstrate on patients in several workshops, and I was greatly influenced in my work with hemiplegia both by her theories and by the superb art of "her hands on techniques."

Nineteen sixty three ended with an interesting comment by Signe. She noted that, "my first social security check arrived. For six months $642."

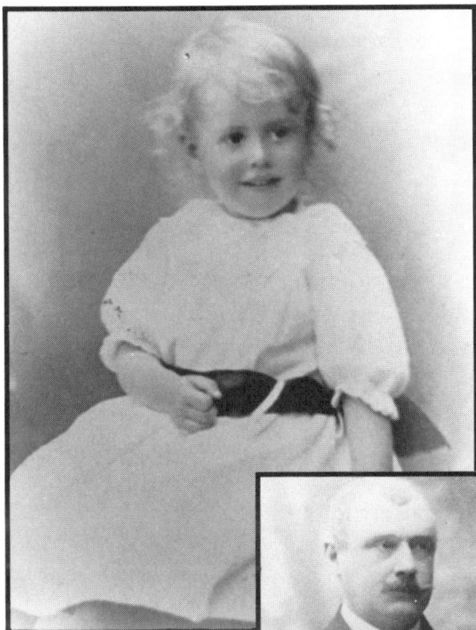

Photo: Signe, age two.

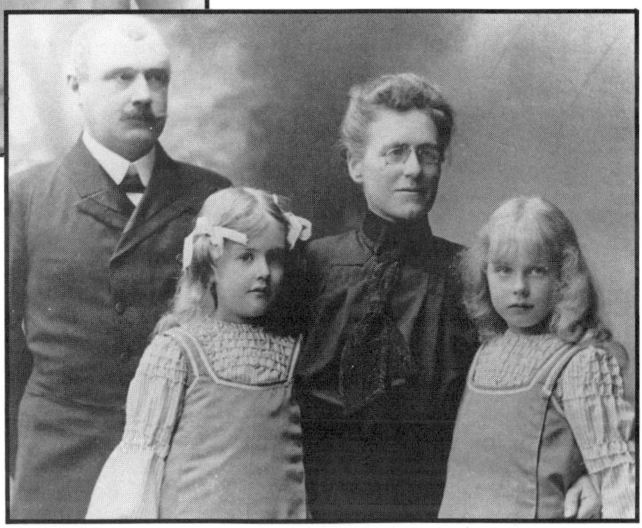

The Brunnstrom Family, 1905.

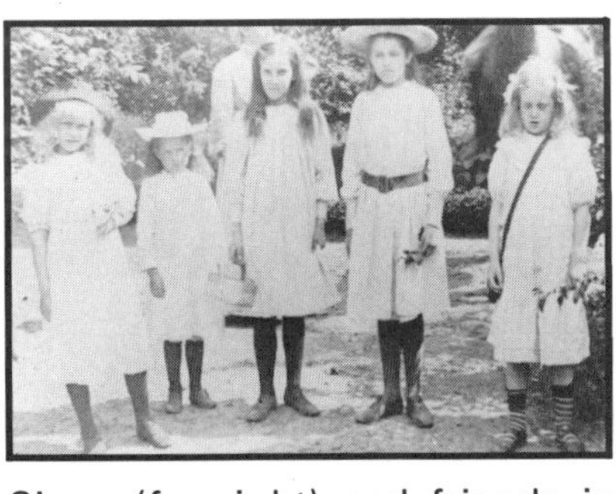

Signe (far right) and friends in Hofdala, 1905.

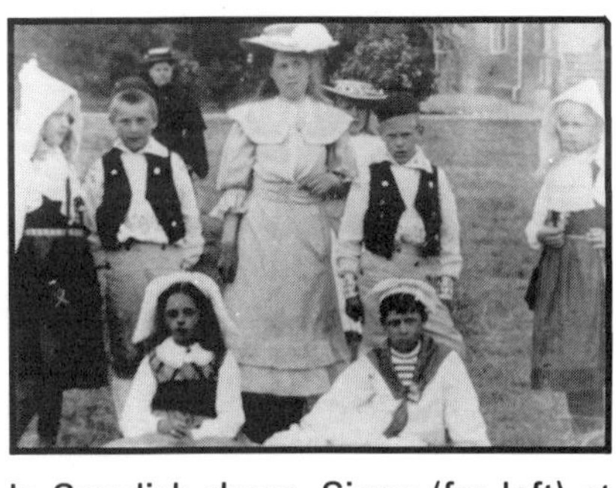

In Swedish dress, Signe (far left) at Bonnely, 1906.

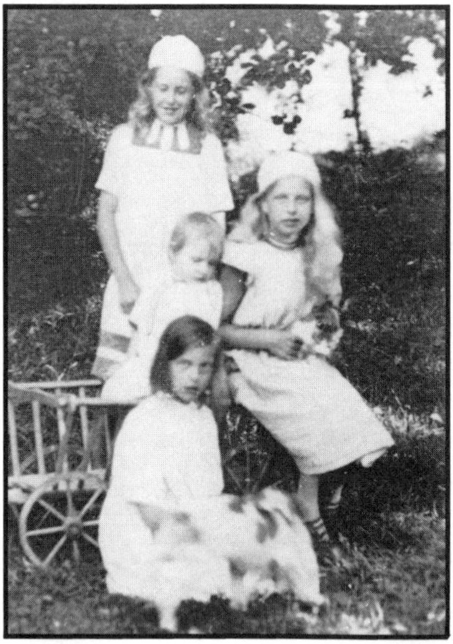

Standing in the rear, Signe in 1908 at Nobbeled.

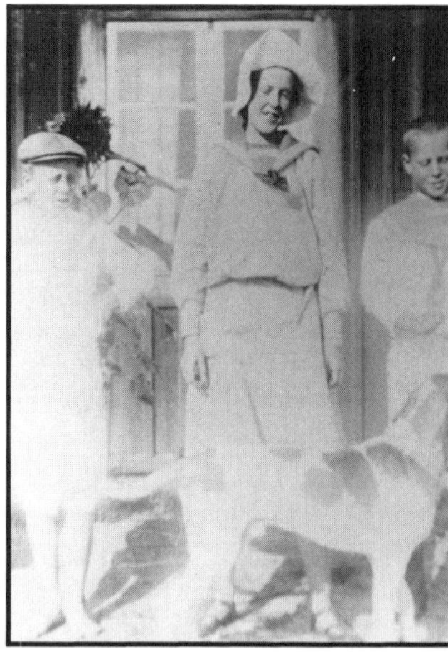

A tall Signe in 1911.

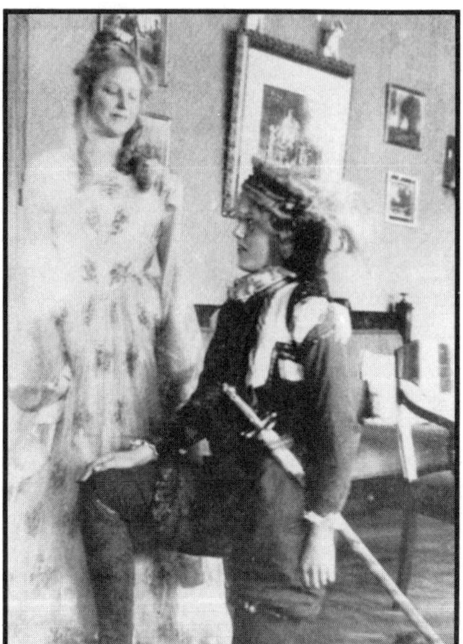

December 1913, Elsa (standing) and Signe in costume for a play.

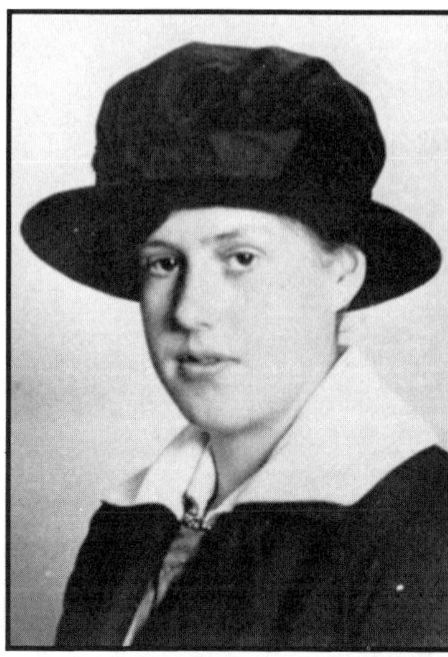

Signe, the serious student, at age 17.

Signe, (second from left) with classmates at Eksjo, 1915.

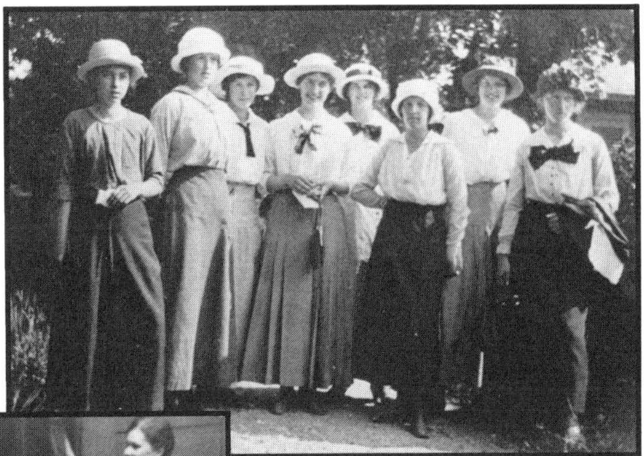

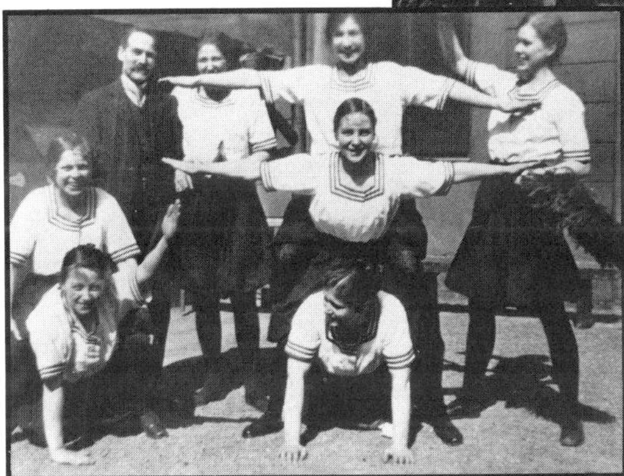

In the physical education gymnastic class, 1918. Signe at far right.

1918, patterns of movement in the gymnastic class. Signe is in the forefront.

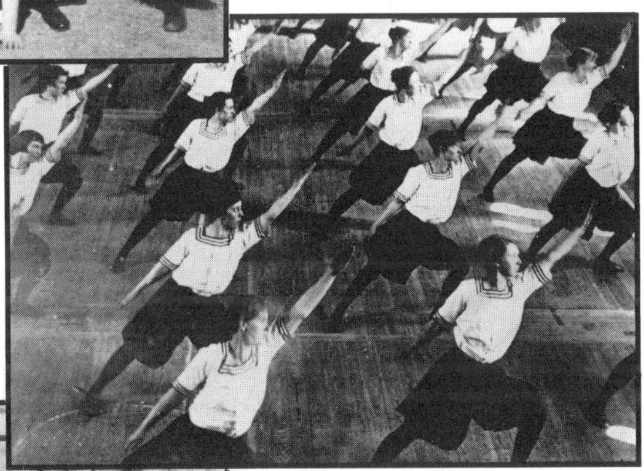

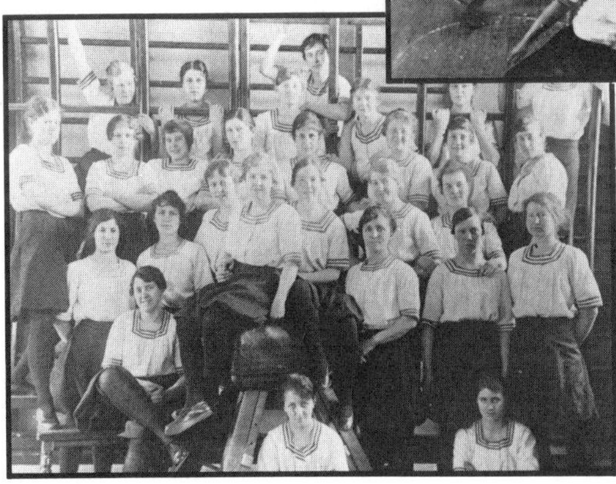

The gymnastic class, 1918. Signe standing at far left with folded arms.

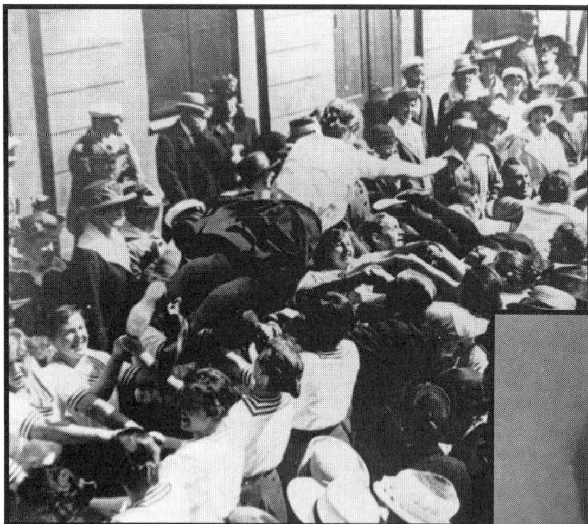

Celebration after passing the "student exam," Stockholm, 1919.

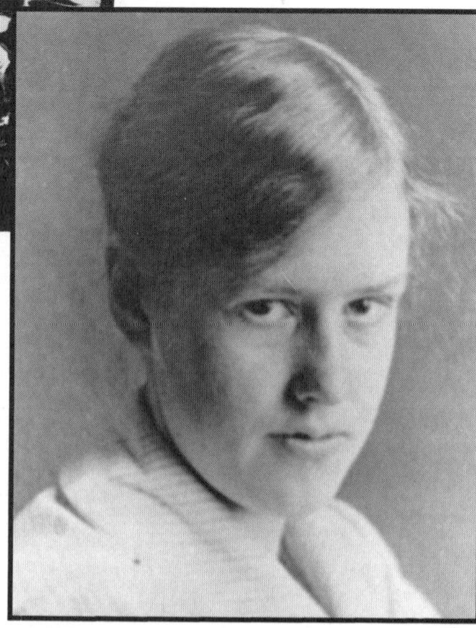

1919.

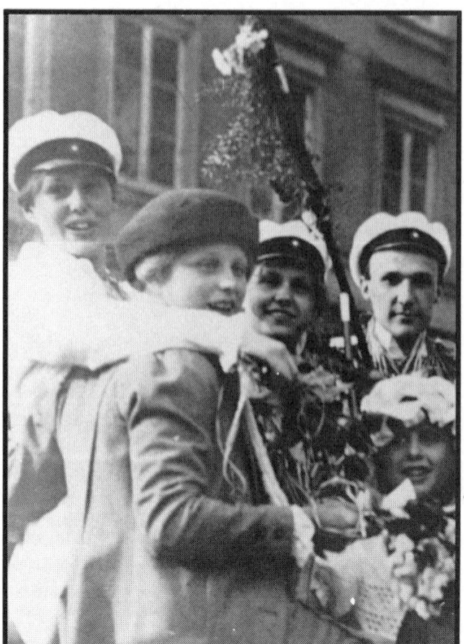

Signe with sister Elsa and two friends after the student exam celebration. Signe's younger sister, Ingegard, is seen at the right.

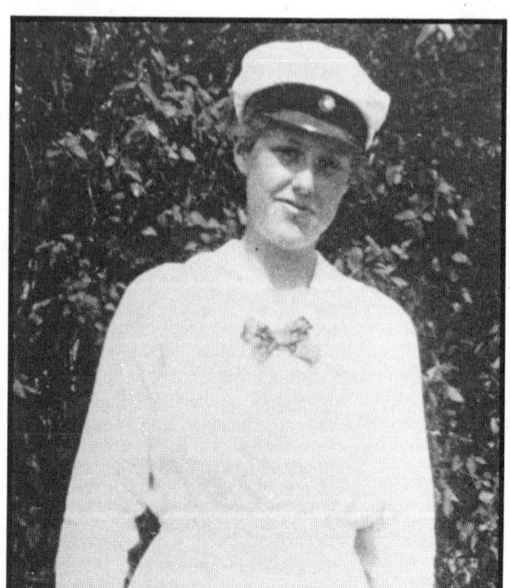

1919

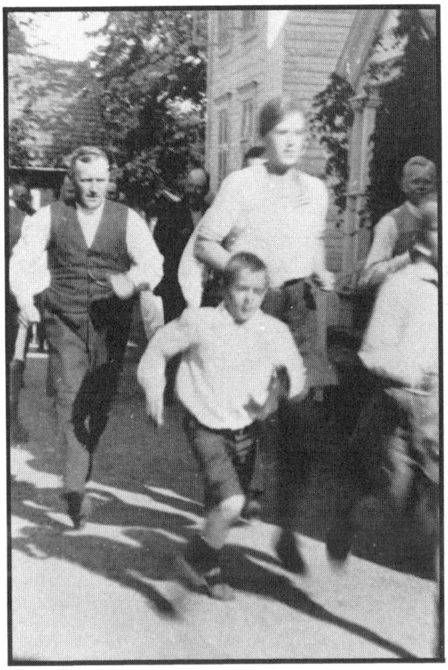

Leading the "porridge run" for fitness.

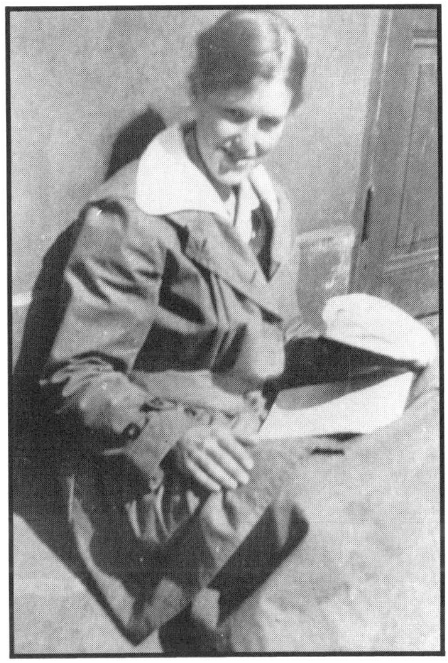

The student in 1919.

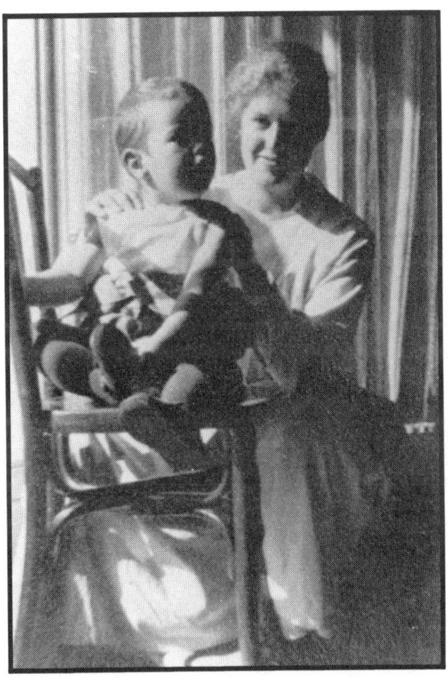

In early 1920, Signe worked with "polio" children in Berne, Switzerland.

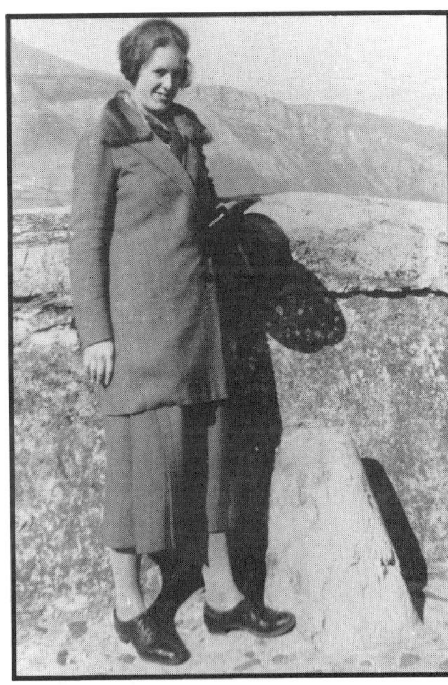

1925, Zurich.

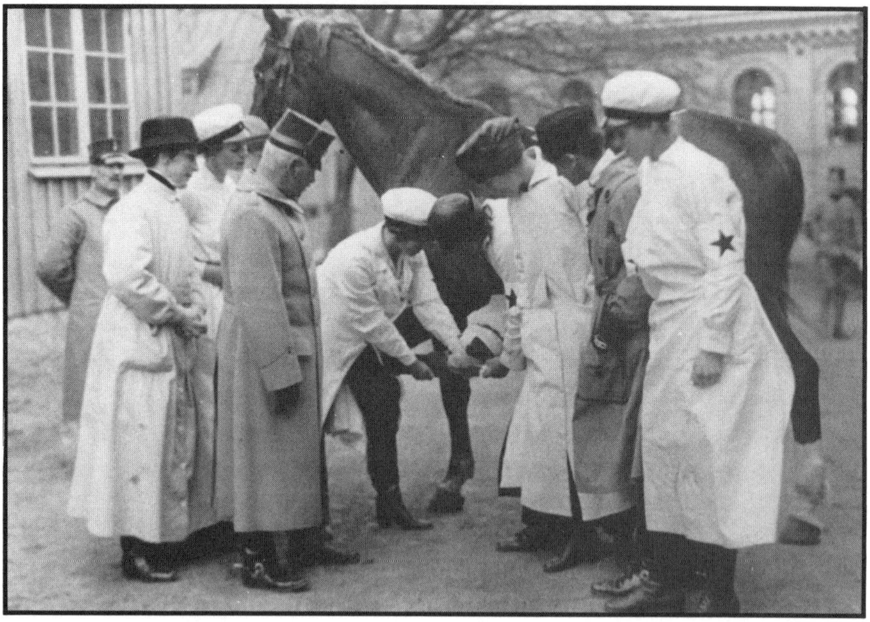

Between 1917-1919 Signe was a member of the Red Star equestrian organization. Signe far right.

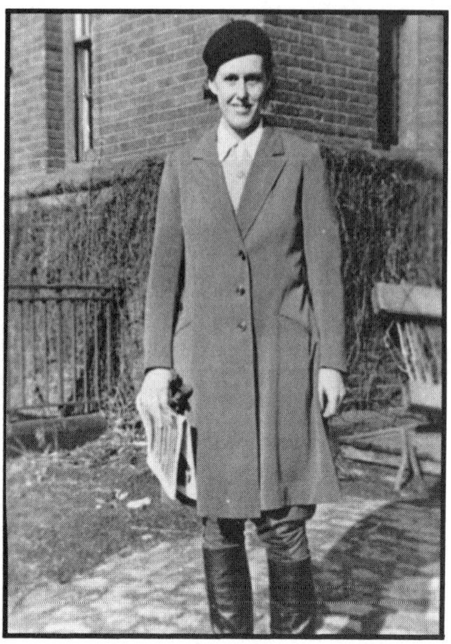

1936, ready for an afternoon of riding.

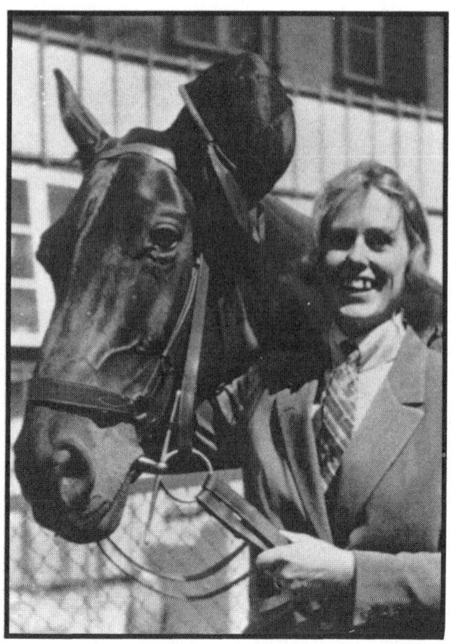

Horseback riding was a favorite activity in 1925 in Lucerne.

Signe, the skier, in 1925.

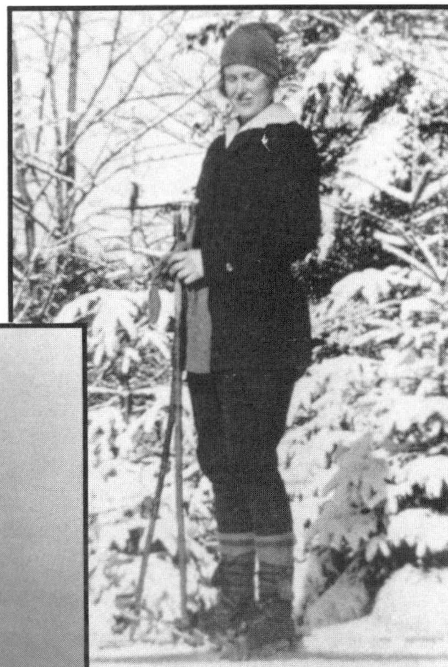

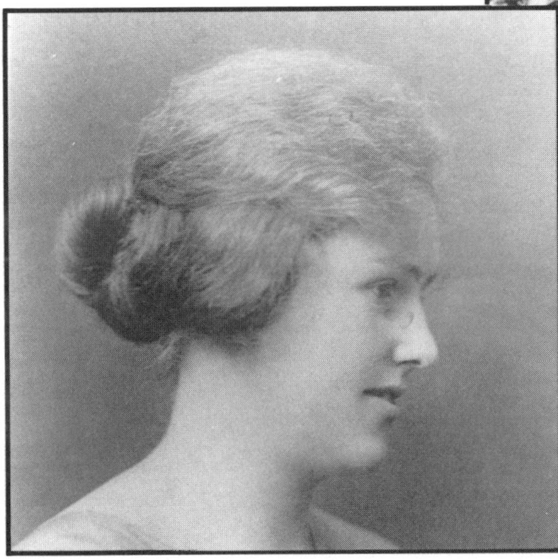

Signe photographed at age 21 in Zurich.

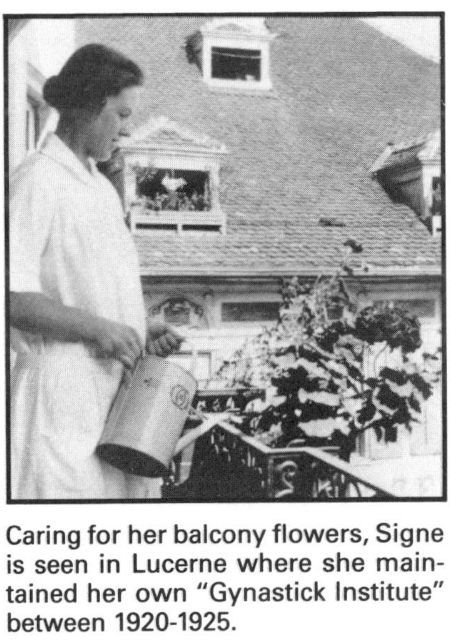

Caring for her balcony flowers, Signe is seen in Lucerne where she maintained her own "Gynastick Institute" between 1920-1925.

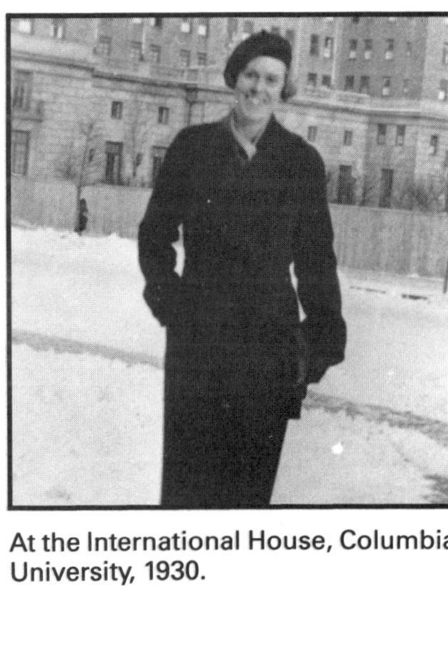

At the International House, Columbia University, 1930.

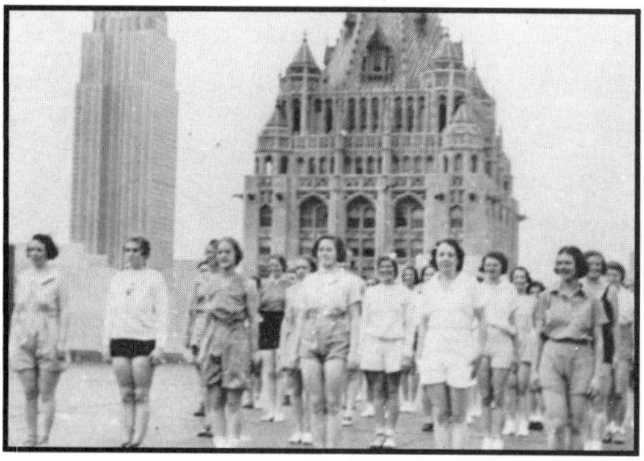

Signe instituted special exercise classes for women on the roof of the Metropolitan Life Insurance Building, New York City, 1941.

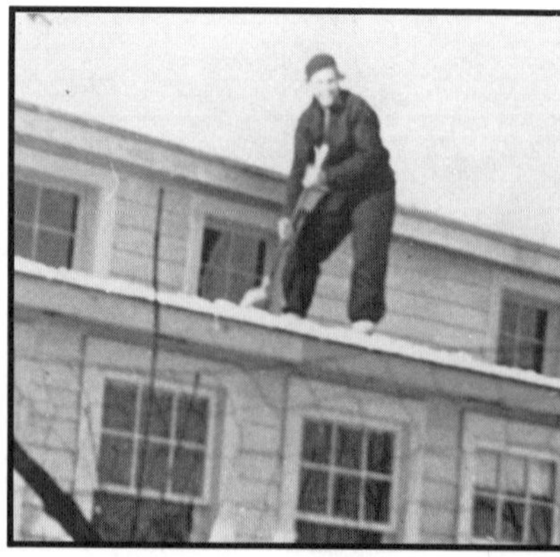

Working on the roof of the "chicken coop" in Carmel, NY, 1941.

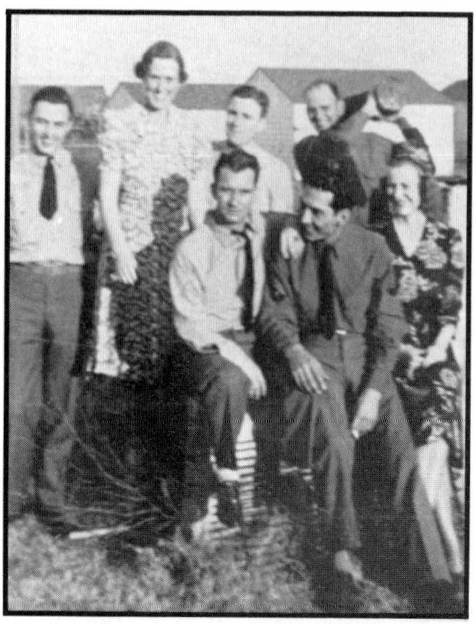

As a civilian physical therapist in 1942, Signe stood above the soldiers in Wichita Falls, Texas.

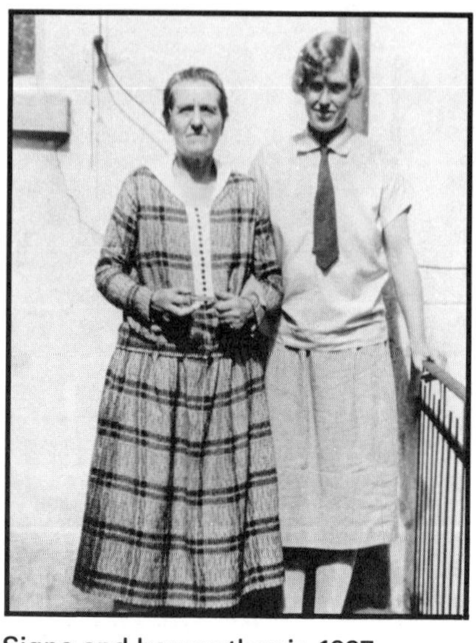

Signe and her mother in 1937.

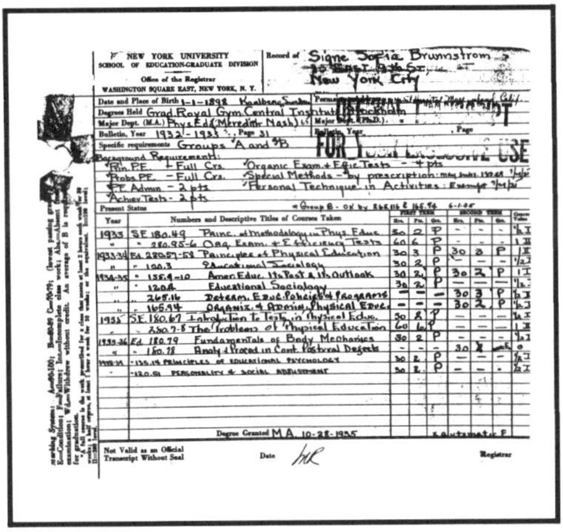

NEW YORK UNIVERSITY
SCHOOL OF EDUCATION-GRADUATE DIVISION
Office of the Registrar
WASHINGTON SQUARE EAST, NEW YORK, N. Y.

Record of Signe Sofia Brunnstrom
New York City

Date and Place of Birth 1-1-1898 Karlberg, Sweden
Degrees Held Grad. Royal Gym. Central Institute Stockholm
Major Dept. (M.A.) Phys. Ed. (Meredith Nash)
Bulletin, Year 1932-1933, Page 31
Specific requirements Groups A and B
Major Dept. (Ph.D.)
Bulletin, Year , Page
OFFICIAL TRANSCRIPT
FOR [illegible] USE

Background Requirements:
Prin. P.E. - Full Crs.
Probs. P.E. - Full Crs.
P.E. Admin - 2 pts
Achiev. Tests - 2 pts
Organic Exam. + Effic. Tests - 4 pts
Special Methods - by prescription [illegible]
Personal Technique in Activities: Exempt [illegible]

Present Status
Group B - OK by 265.16 & 165.94 6-1-35

Year	Numbers and Descriptive Titles of Courses Taken	First Term Hrs.	First Term Pts.	First Term Gr.	Second Term Hrs.	Second Term Pts.	Second Term Gr.	Course Value
1933	SE 180.49 Princ. of Methodology in Phys. Educ.	30	2	P	-	-	-	½ I
"	" 280.95-6 Org. Exam. + Efficiency Tests	60	6	P	-	-	-	1 II
1933-34	Ed. 280.57-58 Principles of Physical Education	30	3	P	30	3	P	1 II
"	" 120.3 Educational Sociology	30	2	P	-	-	-	½ I
1934-35	" 135.9-10 Amer. Educ. Its Past & Its Outlook	30	2	P	30	2	P	1 I
"	" 120A Educational Sociology	30	2	P	—	—	—	½ I
"	" 265.16 Determ. Educ. Policies of Programs	—	—	—	30	3	P	½ I
"	" 165.94 Organiz. & Admin. Physical Educ.	—	—	—	30	2	P	½ I
1935	S.E. 180.67 Introduction to Tests in Physical Educ.	30	2	P	—	—	—	½ I
"	" 280.7-8 The Problems of Physical Education	60	6	P	—	—	—	1 II
1935-36	Ed. 180.79 Fundamentals of Body Mechanics	30	2	P	-	-	-	½ I
"	" 180.78 Analy. & Proced. in Cont. Postural Defects	-	-	-	30	[illegible]	[illegible]	0
1938-39	" 135.14 Principles of Educational Psychology	30	2	P	—	—	—	½ I
"	" 120.51 Personality & Social Adjustment	30	2	P	—	—	-	½ I

Degree Granted M.A. 10-28-1935

Not Valid as an Official Transcript Without Seal
Date
Registrar

Signe's transcript from New York University, New York, New York.

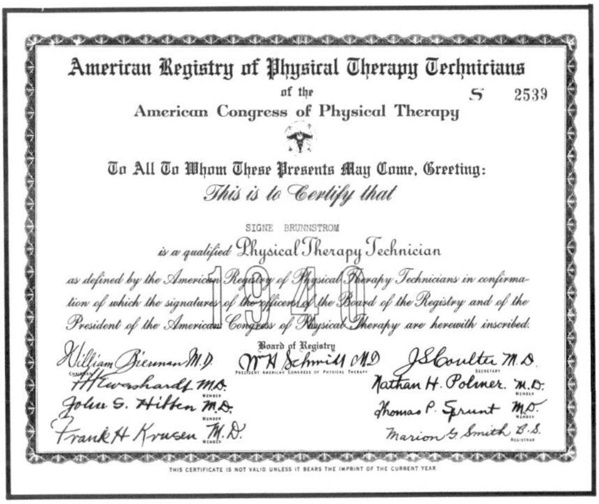

American Registry of Physical Therapy Technicians
of the
American Congress of Physical Therapy
S 2539

To All To Whom These Presents May Come, Greeting:
This is to Certify that

SIGNE BRUNNSTROM

is a qualified Physical Therapy Technician
as defined by the American Registry of Physical Therapy Technicians in confirmation of which the signatures of the officers of the Board of the Registry and of the President of the American Congress of Physical Therapy are herewith inscribed.

1940

Board of Registry

William Bierman M.D. — Chairman
W. H. Schmidt M.D. — President American Congress of Physical Therapy
J. S. Coulter M.D. — Secretary
H. Ewerhardt M.D.
Nathan H. Polmer M.D. — Member
John S. Hibben M.D. — Member
Thomas P. Sprunt M.D. — Member
Frank H. Krusen M.D. — Member
Marion G. Smith B.S. — Registrar

THIS CERTIFICATE IS NOT VALID UNLESS IT BEARS THE IMPRINT OF THE CURRENT YEAR

Certificate from the American Registry of Physical Therapy Technicians, 1940.

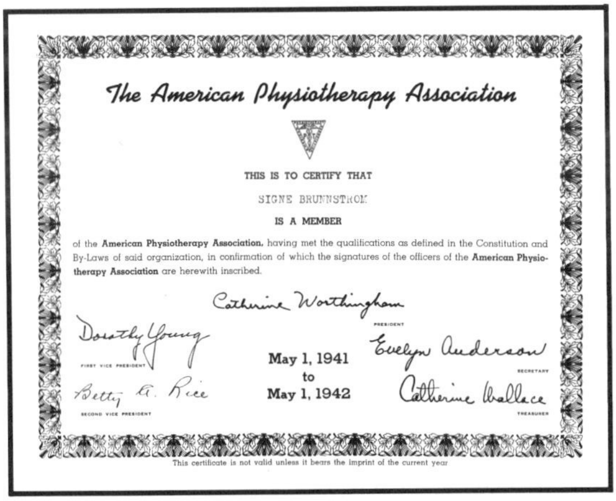

The American Physiotherapy Association

THIS IS TO CERTIFY THAT

SIGNE BRUNNSTROM

IS A MEMBER

of the **American Physiotherapy Association**, having met the qualifications as defined in the Constitution and By-Laws of said organization, in confirmation of which the signatures of the officers of the **American Physiotherapy Association** are herewith inscribed.

Catherine Worthingham — President
Dorothy Young — First Vice President
Betty A. Rice — Second Vice President
Evelyn Anderson — Secretary
Catherine Wallace — Treasurer

May 1, 1941
to
May 1, 1942

This certificate is not valid unless it bears the imprint of the current year

1941 certificate from the American Physiotherapy Association.

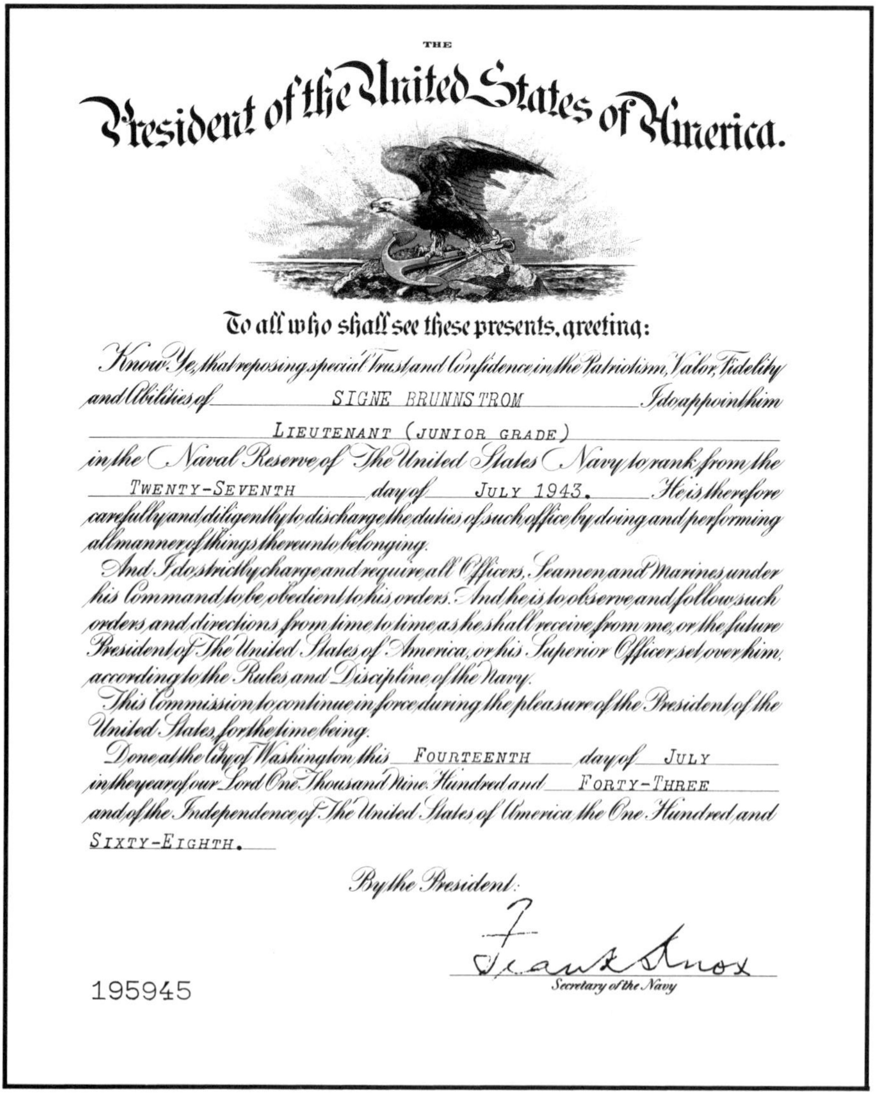

THE

President of the United States of America.

To all who shall see these presents, greeting:

Know Ye, that reposing special Trust and Confidence in the Patriotism, Valor, Fidelity and Abilities of SIGNE BRUNNSTROM I do appoint him LIEUTENANT (JUNIOR GRADE) in the Naval Reserve of The United States Navy to rank from the TWENTY-SEVENTH day of JULY 1943. He is therefore carefully and diligently to discharge the duties of such office by doing and performing all manner of things thereunto belonging.

And I do strictly charge and require all Officers, Seamen and Marines under his Command to be obedient to his orders. And he is to observe and follow such orders and directions from time to time as he shall receive from me, or the future President of The United States of America, or his Superior Officer set over him, according to the Rules and Discipline of the Navy.

This Commission to continue in force during the pleasure of the President of the United States, for the time being.

Done at the City of Washington this FOURTEENTH day of JULY in the year of our Lord One Thousand Nine Hundred and FORTY-THREE and of the Independence of The United States of America the One Hundred and SIXTY-EIGHTH.

By the President:

Frank Knox
Secretary of the Navy

195945

Signe's Commission to the Rank of Lieutenant (Junior Grade) 1943.

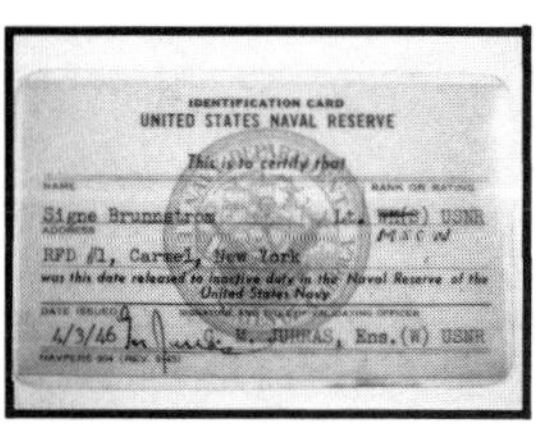

IDENTIFICATION CARD
UNITED STATES NAVAL RESERVE

This is to certify that

Signe Brunnstrom Lt. ~~W(R)~~ USNR

RFD #1, Carmel, New York

was this date released to inactive duty in the Naval Reserve of the United States Navy

4/3/46 G. M. JURRAS, Ens.(W) USNR

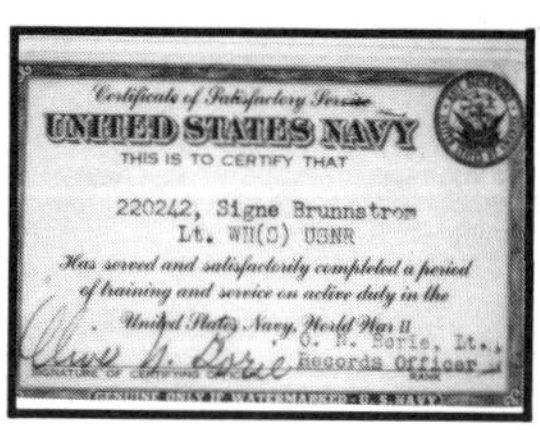

Certificate of Satisfactory Service
UNITED STATES NAVY
THIS IS TO CERTIFY THAT

220242, Signe Brunnstrom
Lt. WR(S) USNR

Has served and satisfactorily completed a period of training and service on active duty in the United States Navy, World War II

O. N. Boric, Lt., Records Officer

Signe's naval identification cards.

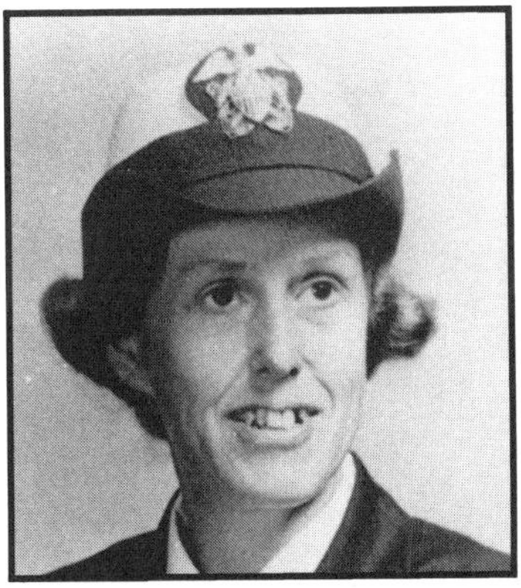

Lt./J.G. Signe Brunnstrom, U.S.N. (photo by Merin-Baliban of Philadelphia) 1945.

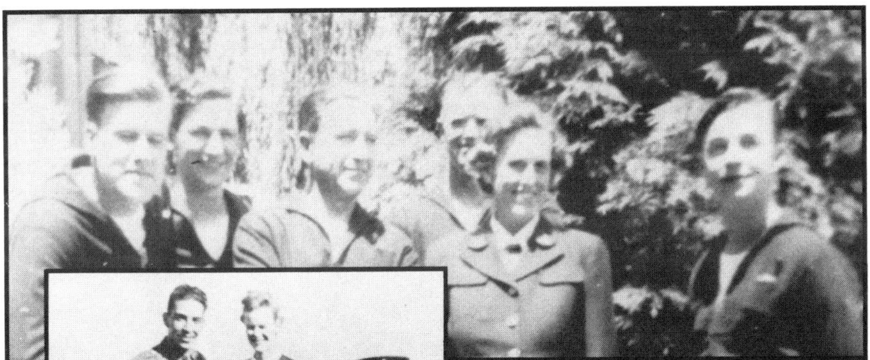

The Physical Therapy staff at Mare Island 1944 with Lt. Brunnstrom. Robert Teckemeyer (left) became Associate Executive Director of the APTA.

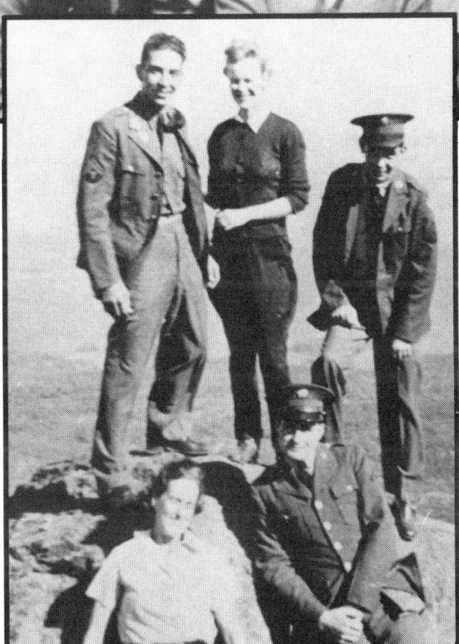

Mary Flickinger (center), Signe's co-worker in the P.T. Department at the army base in Wichita Falls, with Signe and some soliders on an afternoon outing, 1942.

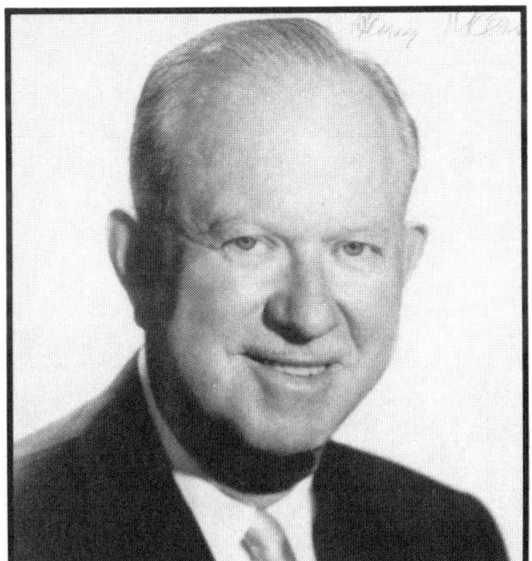

Dr. Henry Kessler.

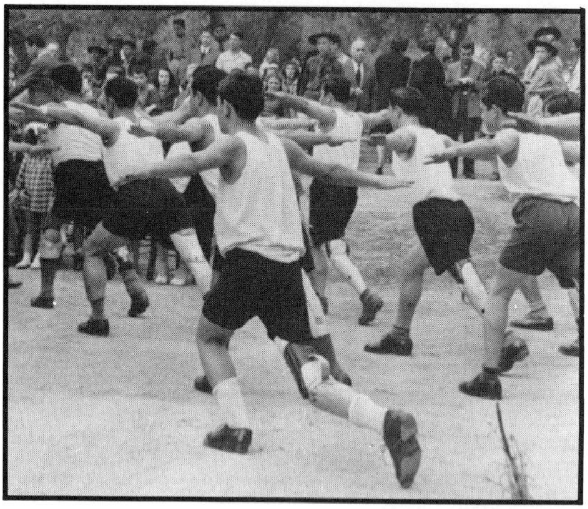

Signe's gymnastic training came in useful in Athens when working with amputees.

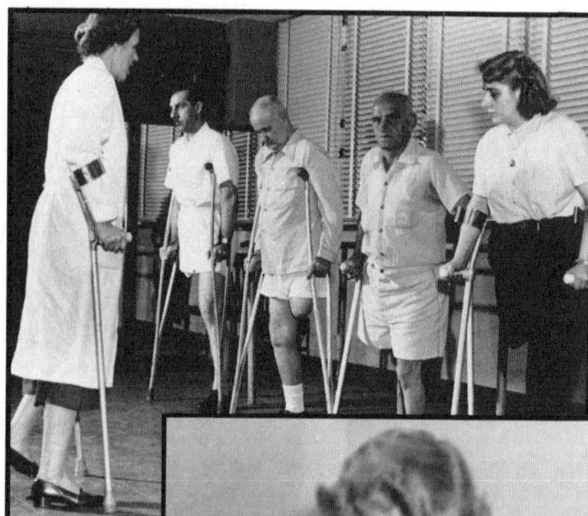

Teaching a class of amputee patients at NYU-IRM, 1956 (Photo by AV Department).

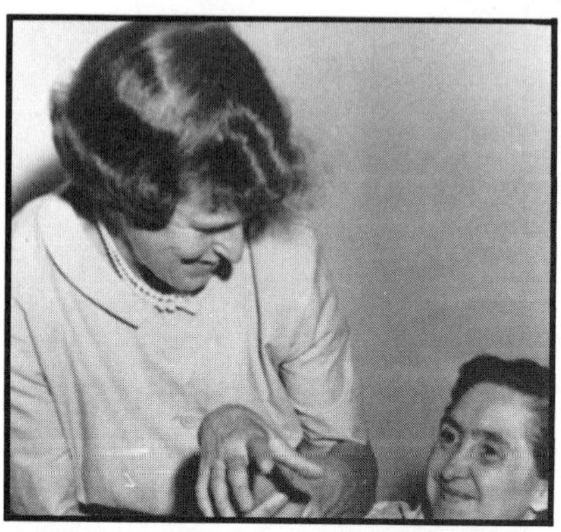

Signe and patient at Kessler Institute, 1952.

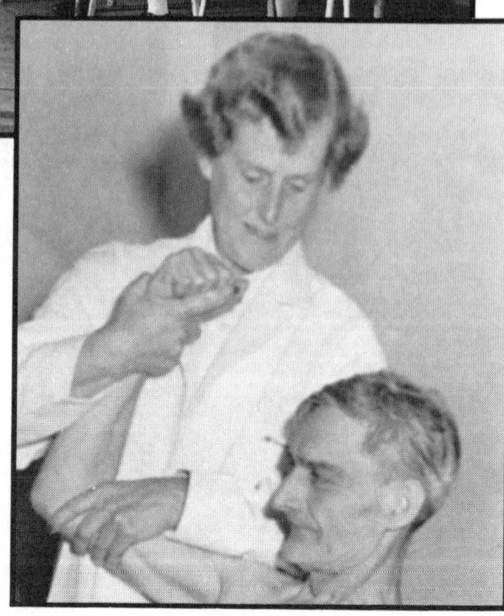

September 1958, Signe demonstrates treatment techniques with a patient from the VA Hospital in Michigan.

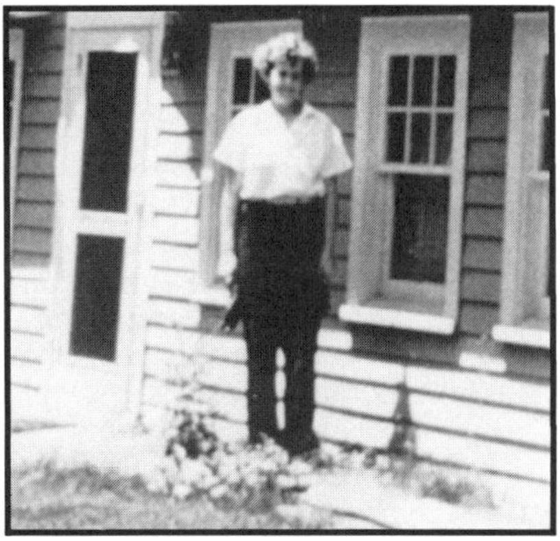

In front of the renovated "chicken coop", 1956.

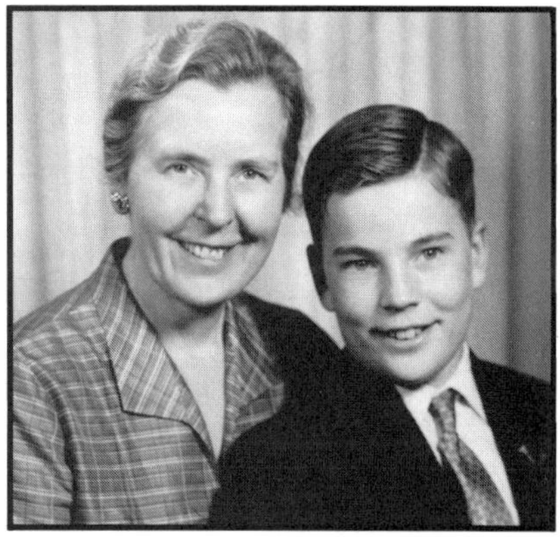

Elfriede Prins and son Robert, 1958.

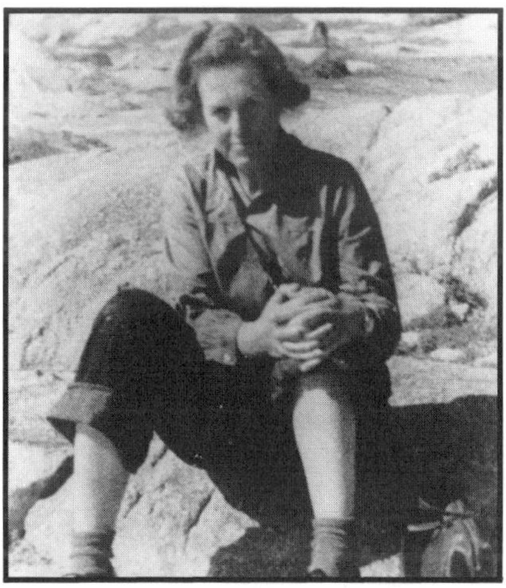

At Mare Island, California, 1947.

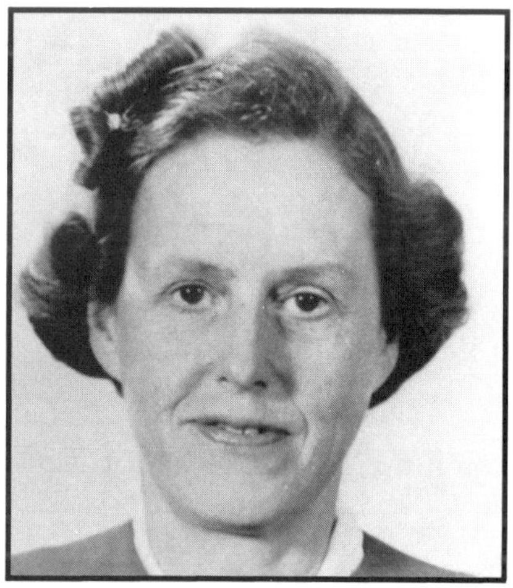

Signe's 1946 passport photo.

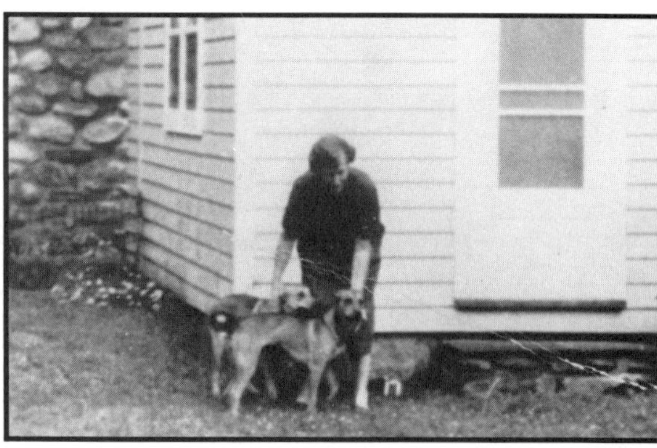

Signe with her two loyal friends, Kaya and Rebel, at home on Bullet Hole Road, Carmel, NY, 1956.

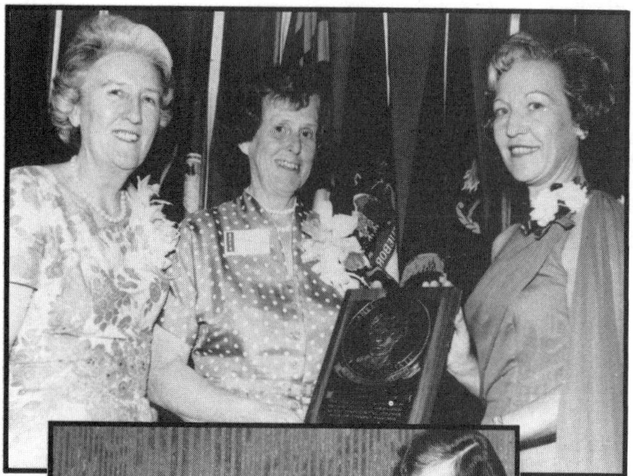

July 1, 1965, Cleveland, Ohio. At the Annual Conference of the American Physical Therapy Association, Ms. Brunnstrom (center) receives Marian Williams Research award with Lucille Daniels (left) Assoc. Editor for APTA, and Mary Elizabeth Kolb, APTA president.

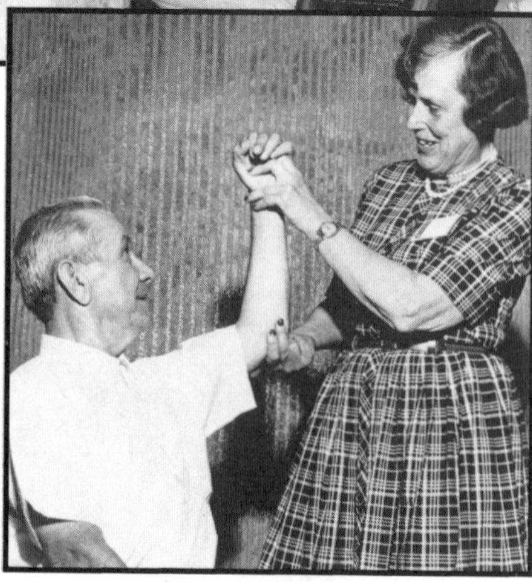

At the APTA Conference, Signe offered a demonstration of treatment techniques.

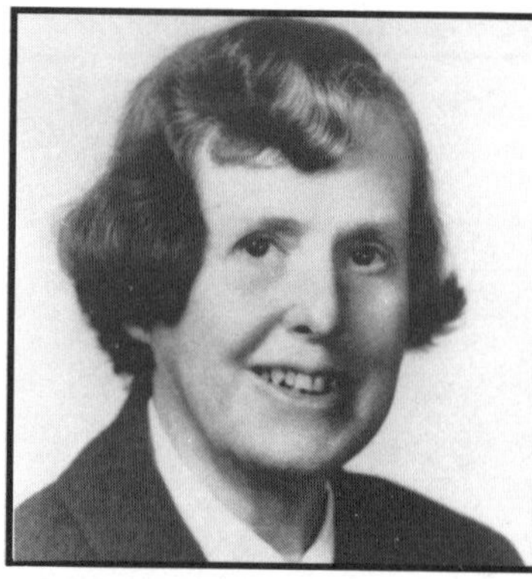

Signe at age 65.

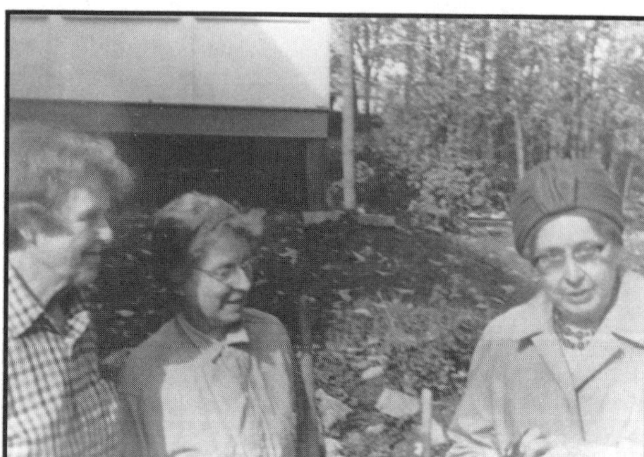

In 1970, sisters Elsa (center) and Ingegerd (right) visited Signe in Carmel, NY.

Doing what she liked best, Signe enjoyed being with the physical therapy students at Stony Brook. Front row: Jacqui Sherman, Vera DeFord, Signe, Roz Fink. Back row: Maryrose Babino and Al Farrago. June 1975.

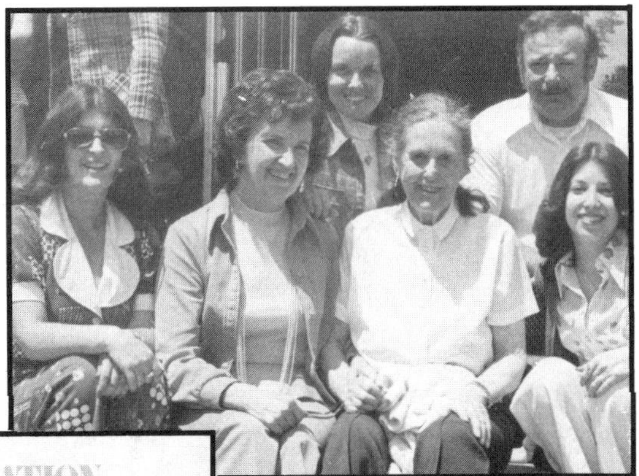

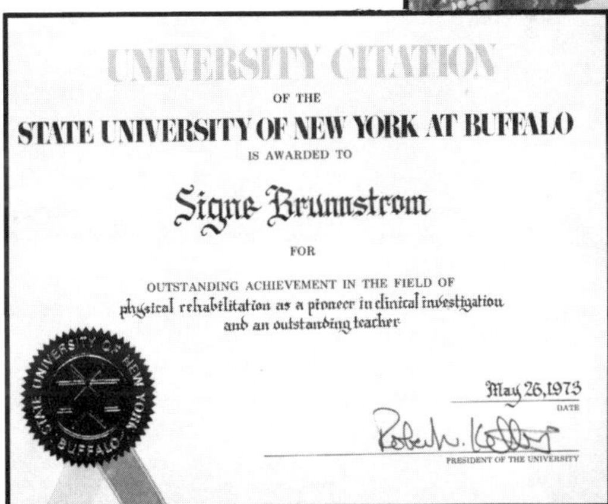

UNIVERSITY CITATION

OF THE

STATE UNIVERSITY OF NEW YORK AT BUFFALO

IS AWARDED TO

Signe Brunnstrom

FOR

OUTSTANDING ACHIEVEMENT IN THE FIELD OF physical rehabilitation as a pioneer in clinical investigation and an outstanding teacher

May 26, 1973
DATE

PRESIDENT OF THE UNIVERSITY

Citation from the State University of New York, Buffalo, 1973.

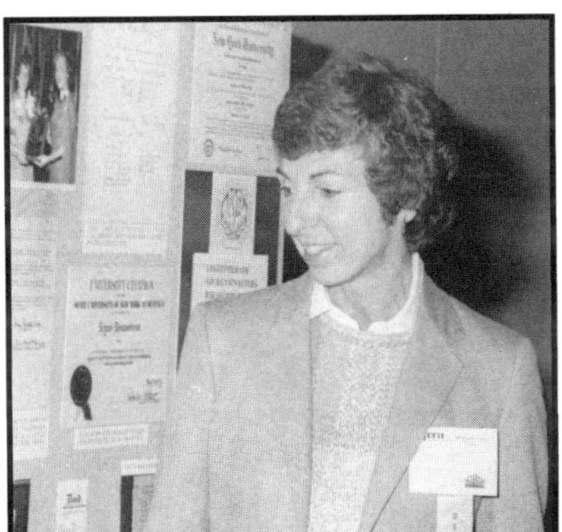

Jeanne LaVigne, a dear friend, continues to teach and promote the "Brunnstrom Approach."

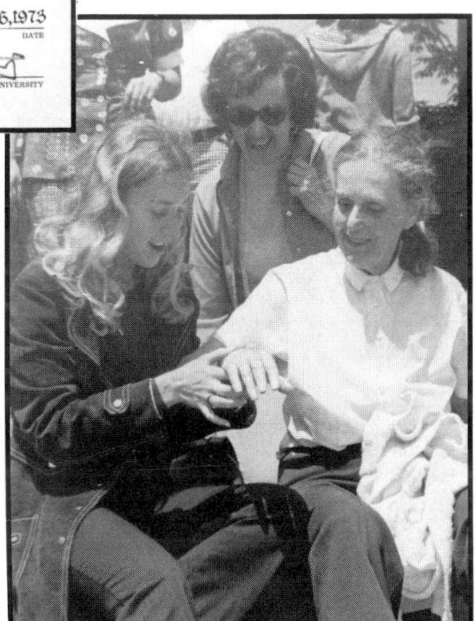

As always, Signe was ready for a lesson even during a break in the workshop. Gayle Edelstein, a senior P.T. student received Signe's cooperation in a demonstration of hand function. Vera DeFord looks on.

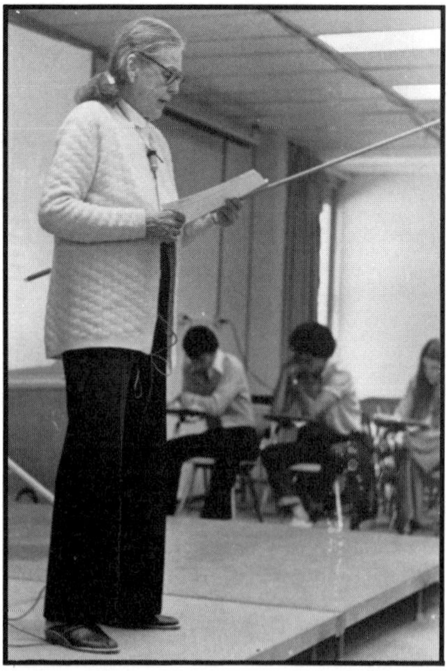

Signe, the instructor at SUNY Stony Brook, June 1975.

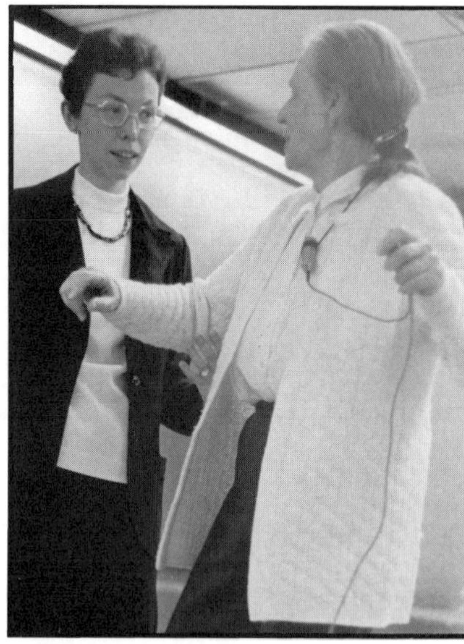

Katherine Sawner of the State University of New York at Buffalo was among Signe's closest friends and supporters. She received the rights to Signe's book, "Movement Therapy in Hemiplegia."

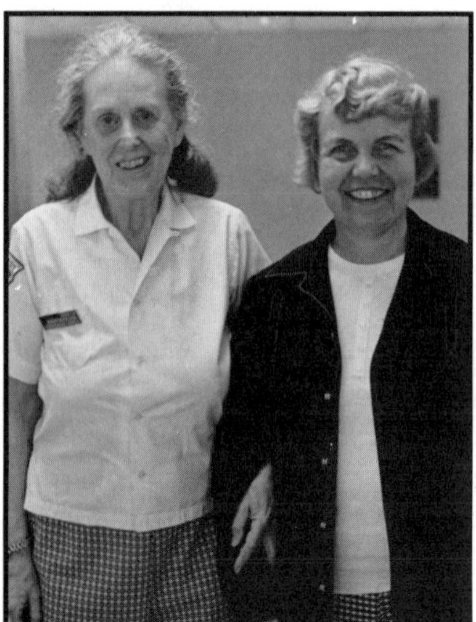

Signe gave the rights to her book, "Clinical Kinesiology" to one of her dearest colleagues, Ruth Dickinson of Columbia University.

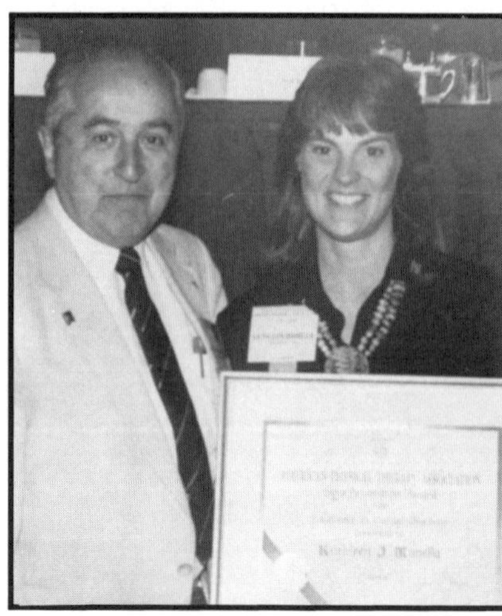

Jay Schleichkorn presented the first Signe Brunnstrom Award for Clinical Excellence to Kathleen Manella of Los Angeles Orthopaedic Hospital, June 1988 at the APTA annual conference in Las Vegas.

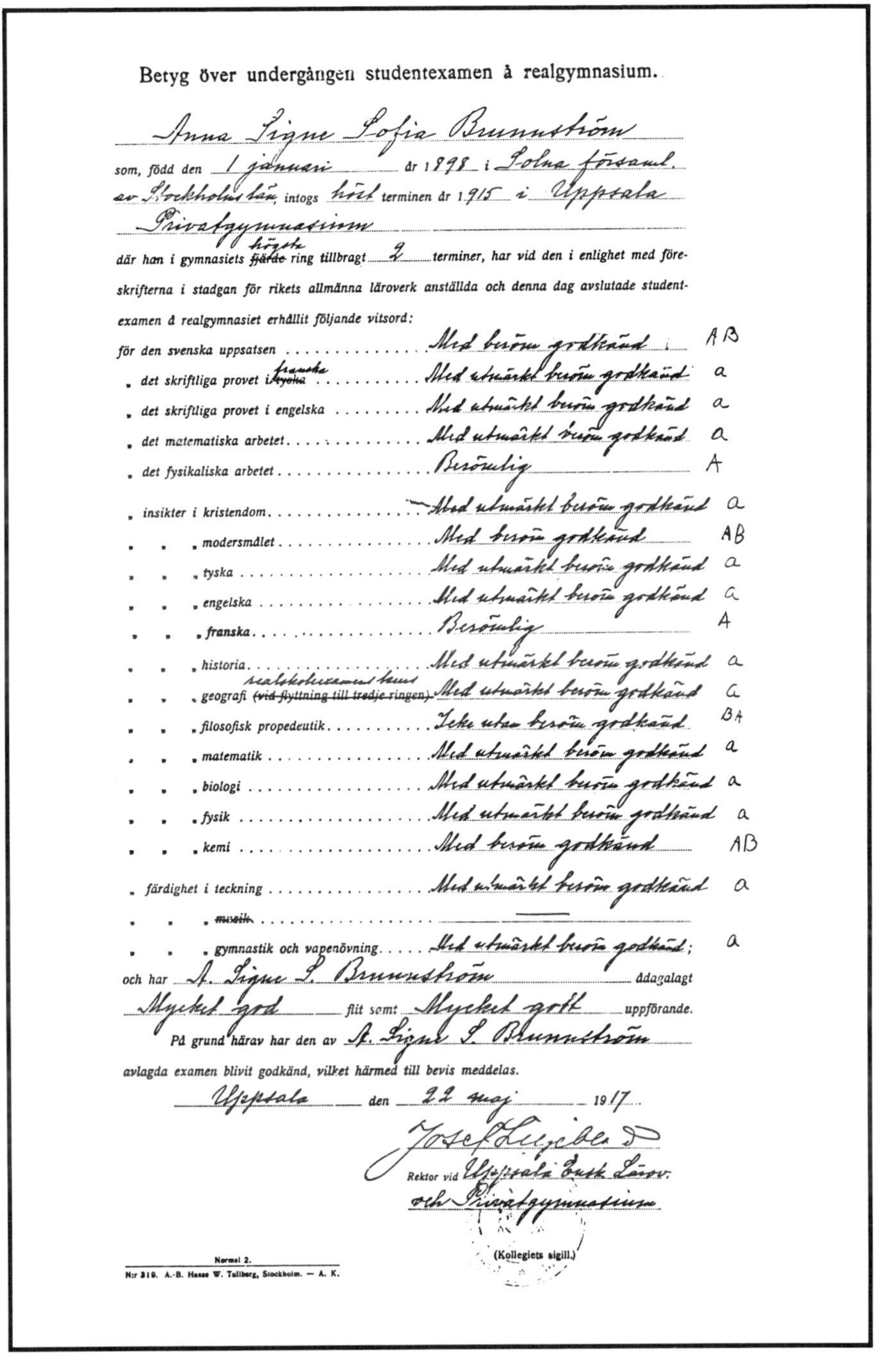

Betyg över undergången studentexamen å realgymnasium.

Anna Signe Sofia Brunnström

som, född den 1 januari år 1898 i Solna församl. av Stockholms län, intogs höst terminen år 1915 i Uppsala Privatgymnasium

där han i gymnasiets ~~fjärde~~ högsta ring tillbragt 2 terminer, har vid den i enlighet med föreskrifterna i stadgan för rikets allmänna läroverk anställda och denna dag avslutade studentexamen å realgymnasiet erhållit följande vitsord:

för den svenska uppsatsen	Med beröm godkänd	AB
„ det skriftliga provet i ~~tyska~~ franska	Med utmärkt beröm godkänd	a
„ det skriftliga provet i engelska	Med utmärkt beröm godkänd	a
„ det matematiska arbetet	Med utmärkt beröm godkänd	a
„ det fysikaliska arbetet	Berömlig	A
„ insikter i kristendom	Med utmärkt beröm godkänd	a
„ „ „ modersmålet	Med beröm godkänd	AB
„ „ „ tyska	Med utmärkt beröm godkänd	a
„ „ „ engelska	Med utmärkt beröm godkänd	a
„ „ „ franska	Berömlig	A
„ „ „ historia	Med utmärkt beröm godkänd	a
„ „ „ geografi ~~(vid flyttning till tredje ringen)~~ realskolexamen lems	Med utmärkt beröm godkänd	a
„ „ „ filosofisk propedeutik	Icke utan beröm godkänd	BA
„ „ „ matematik	Med utmärkt beröm godkänd	a
„ „ „ biologi	Med utmärkt beröm godkänd	a
„ „ „ fysik	Med utmärkt beröm godkänd	a
„ „ „ kemi	Med beröm godkänd	AB
„ färdighet i teckning	Med utmärkt beröm godkänd	a
„ „ „ ~~musik~~	—	
„ „ „ gymnastik och vapenövning	Med utmärkt beröm godkänd;	a

och har A. Signe S. Brunnström ådagalagt Mycket god flit samt Mycket gott uppförande.

På grund härav har den av A. Signe S. Brunnström avlagda examen blivit godkänd, vilket härmed till bevis meddelas.

Uppsala den 22 maj 1917.

Josef Lagerblad
Rektor vid Uppsala Enskl. Läroverk och Privatgymnasium

(Kollegiets sigill.)

Normal 2.
N:r 319. A.-B. Hasse W. Tullberg, Stockholm. — A. K.

Signe's report card, Uppsala College, 1917.

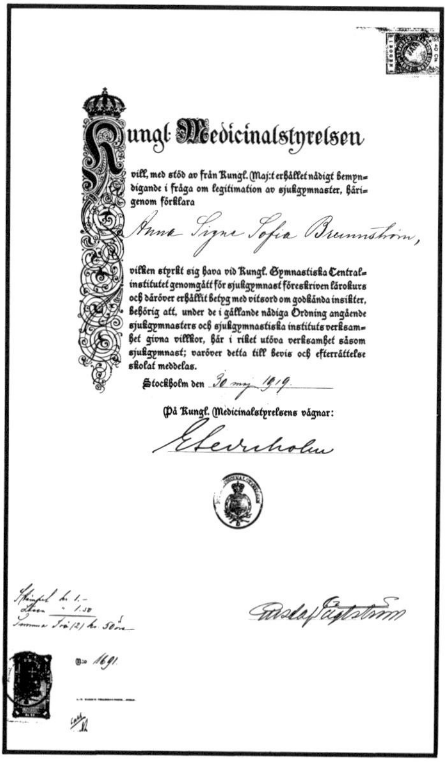

Kungl. Medicinalstyrelsen

vill, med stöd av från Kungl. Maj:t erhållet nådigt bemyndigande i fråga om legitimation av sjukgymnaster, härigenom förklara

Anna Signe Sofia Brunnström,

vilken styrkt sig hava vid Kungl. Gymnastiska Centralinstitutet genomgått för sjukgymnast föreskriven lärokurs och däröver erhållit betyg med vitsord om godkända insikter, behörig att, under de i gällande nådiga Ordning angående sjukgymnasters och sjukgymnastiska instituts verksamhet givna villkor, här i riket utöva verksamhet såsom sjukgymnast; varöver detta till bevis och efterrättelse skolat meddelas.

Stockholm den 30 maj 1919.

På Kungl. Medicinalstyrelsens vägnar:

No 1691

Graduation diploma, 30 May, 1919.

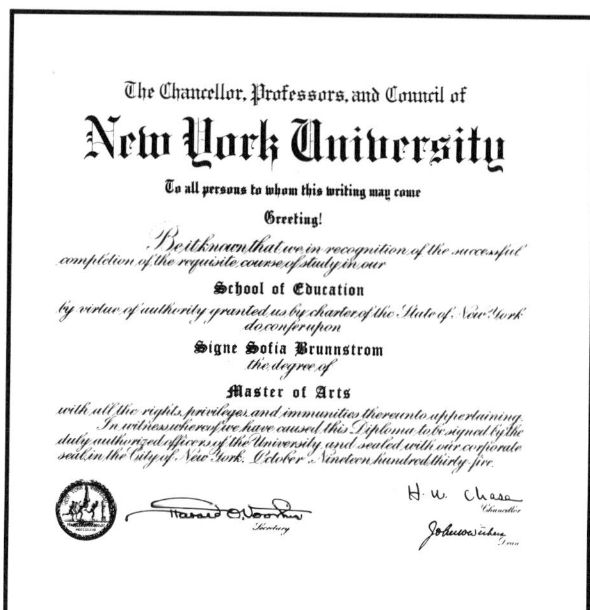

The Chancellor, Professors, and Council of

New York University

To all persons to whom this writing may come

Greeting!

Be it known that we in recognition of the successful completion of the requisite course of study in our

School of Education

by virtue of authority granted us by charter of the State of New York do confer upon

Signe Sofia Brunnstrom

the degree of

Master of Arts

with all the rights, privileges, and immunities thereunto appertaining. In witness whereof we have caused this Diploma to be signed by the duly authorized officers of the University and sealed with our corporate seal in the City of New York, October Nineteen hundred thirty-five.

Secretary

H. W. Chase
Chancellor

Dean

Diploma, New York University, 1935.

Muscle Group Testing

Signe Brunnstrom, M.A.

The importance of accurately measuring muscle strength in the aftercare of infantile paralysis is obvious. To perform an extensive and time consuming muscle test at the beginning of the treatment and at regular intervals afterwards is just so much waste of time unless the test possesses a reasonable amount of accuracy. The purpose of this paper is to give a critical evaluation of the muscle test most commonly used today, pointing out its shortcomings and discussing ways and means of improving it.

Dr. Robert Lovett of Boston and his assistant, Miss Wilhelmina Wright, tried out various methods of testing and recording muscular strength[1]. At first the charts developed by Dr. E. A. Sharpe of Buffalo were used. These charts consisted of drawings of anterior and posterior views of the body with an outline of the most important muscles. The wholly paralyzed muscles were closely shaded, the partially paralyzed muscles were shaded with coarse lines and the normal muscles were not shaded at all. The charts were practical because one glance at the chart would give an approximate idea of the extent of paralysis present. However, "partially paralyzed muscles" would include all muscles which were partially affected, whether the affection were slight or severe. It soon was found that a more detailed record of the affected muscles was necessary.

The "Spring Balance Muscle Test," worked out by E. G. Martin of the Physiological Department of the Harvard Medical School in cooperation with Lovett and described in various books and articles[1, 2, 3] was a definite improvement on the previous test. By means of this test, gain and loss in muscular strength could be measured in pounds. It proved to be a very reliable test for strong and fairly strong muscle groups. However, extremely weak muscles could not be tested accurately.

The grading system which was finally found most satisfactory by Lovett, and which was soon widely accepted by physicians and technicians, judges the strength of muscles mainly in relation to gravity. Lovett states that "the method of examination described is not a mathematically accurate one, but it has the advantage of requiring no apparatus and of providing a graded series of tests for estimating muscular power.

"The muscles were graded as:

1. Normal.

2. Good, when the muscle was strong enough to overcome gravity and some resistance but was not quite of normal strength.

3. Fair, when the muscle was able to overcome gravity and could perform part of the normal movement.

4. Poor, when slight movement could be accomplished but gravity could not be overcome.

5. Trace, when no movement of the limb could be accomplished but the muscle could be felt to contract.

6. Totally paralyzed, when attempted voluntary movement was not accompanied by any perceptible contraction of the muscle."[1, 4]

This method, or a modification of it, is commonly used in hospitals and clinics today. To these original grades most examiners add pluses and minuses in order to make finer differentiations. Each technician, or each hospital, has a somewhat different interpretation of the grades. The range of motion which can be performed, the number of times a movement can be repeated without causing fatigue or the amount of manual resistance given by the examiner determine the grade. Kendall[5] lists fourteen grades, beginning with "zero" and ending with "normal plus," and also suggests recording muscle strength in percentage to correspond with the above grades. Lowman[6] lists ten different grades, using numerals from 0 to 9. There is no uniformity in testing methods or in terms used. For instance, "fair plus" is described by Lowman as "beginning action of joints but not against gravity or enough to overcome friction of table." Kendall, on the other hand, states that a "fair plus" muscle "completes the arc of motion against gravity and a minimum amount of resistance." What terms are used may not be important in themselves, as long as all individuals in the same institution know their meanings, but it is very confusing to students and to all persons who consult the literature. Standardization of terms, therefore, is highly desirable.

10 East 9th Street, New York, N. Y.

Muscle Group Testing, The Physiotherapy Review, Vol. 21, No. 1, 1941, Reprinted with permission.

PHYSICAL THERAPY IN AFTERCARE OF AMPUTATIONS OF LOWER EXTREMITY

SIGNE BRUNNSTROM
Lieutenant, junior grade W-V(S) (H) U.S.N.R.

At a recent meeting of allied surgeons in Toronto, Canada (February 1944), four "sites of election" were agreed upon as producing satisfactory stumps:

1. *Syme's*—a transmalleolar amputation. To cover the amputation surface, a posterior skin flap which includes the fatty subcutaneous tissue of the heel is utilized. This gives a good end-bearing stump.

2. *Midleg*—an amputation through the middle third of the leg about six inches below the knee. In all midleg amputations the fibula is retained although it is cut shorter than the tibia. Longer stumps are to be avoided, since such stumps usually have poor circulation, are sensitive, and are hard to fit with a prosthesis. Shorter stumps, through the upper third of the leg, are unsatisfactory because they do not provide sufficient leverage for knee action.

3. *Stokes-Gritti*—the femoral condyles are removed and the patella is fused to the end of the femur. It gives a good weight-bearing surface.

4. *Midthigh*—the ideal site is at the junction of the middle and lower third of the femur, although a true midthigh amputation is also quite satisfactory. Amputations through the upper third of the femur do not give as good results. In midthigh amputations skin flaps (but no muscular tissue) are used to cover the end of the stump.[1]

PHYSICAL THERAPY MODALITIES

Heat in some form is often used to improve circulation of the stump and to relieve pain. For circulatory effects contrast baths are particularly recommended. The contrast bath by producing an alternate vasodilatation and vasoconstriction has a more beneficial effect on the circulation than has the hot or warm bath. As a rule long periods of water treatment should be avoided, since they tend to soften the skin. (The skin should be toughened rather than softened.)

[1] Disapproved: Disarticulation of hip; disarticulation of knee; any amputation through the tarsal bones, leaving only the calcaneus and the astragalus, which invariably causes equinus position of the stump.

United States Naval Medical Bulletin, October 1944, Vol. 43, No. 4.

Comparative Strength of Muscles with Similar Function:

A Study on Peripheral Nerve Injuries of the Upper Extremity

Signe Brunnstrom, Lt., U.S.N.R.

By observing the motor dysfunction which appears as a result of injuries to specific peripheral nerves, a considerable amount of information as to relative strength and importance of individual muscles may be obtained. Obviously such studies cannot be carried out on individuals with intact nerve supply, since normally all nerves and muscles function as an integrated whole and not as separate units.

This paper deals with motor dysfunction as observed in cases of paralysis of the spinal accessory, the long thoracic, the axillary, the suprascapular and the musculocutaneous nerves.

Spinal Accessory Nerve

The result of loss of the nerve supply to the trapezius muscle is seen in Figures 1-A—1-D. In the relaxed standing position, the scapula is somewhat downwardly rotated with the inferior angle closer to the spinal column than the superior angle. The entire scapula is lower than on the unaffected side (Fig. 1-A).

During abduction of the arm, the scapulohumeral rhythm is disturbed, but the arm can be abducted without difficulty (Fig. 1-B), the serratus magnus giving satisfactory fixation to the scapula. Arm raising over head is performed with ease (Fig. 1-C), the serratus rotating the scapula. Adduction of the shoulder blades (Fig. 1-D) shows the trapezius contracting vigorously on the left side and missing on the right side. As a whole, there is practically no disability as far as strength and range of motion of abduction is concerned.

Long Thoracic Nerve

With the serratus magnus out of function, the scapula is very unstable. In the relaxed standing position the scapula is "tipped" forward, causing the inferior angle to protrude (Fig. 2-A). The scapula lacks fixation in all motions involving abduction and flexion of the humerus. When the subject places his hand on the opposite shoulder, the vertebral border of the scapula protrudes (Fig. 2-B). Flexion or abduction beyond the horizontal is impossible (Figures 2-C, 2-D). The trapezius can be seen contracting vigorously giving some fixation to the scapula, but without the aid of the serratus it is unable to upward rotate the scapula.

A serratus paralysis causes by far a more serious disability than a trapezius paralysis. These observations confirm previous more detailed studies by this author on the same object.[1]

Axillary Nerve Paralysis

Until recently it has been assumed that the deltoid muscle is the most important muscle in abduction of the arm. Bowen[2] calls the deltoid the large abductor and the supraspinatus a "small associate." He further states that "Loss of one or more of the three portions of the deltoid interferes so seriously with all movements involving elevation of the arm that subjects with this defect have much difficulty in feeding and dressing themselves. Loss of the posterior

U. S. Naval Hospital, Mare Island, Calif.

The opinions expressed in this article are those of the writer personally and are in no way the official expression of the Medical Department of the U. S. Navy.

Reprinted from the Physiotherapy Review (Vol. 26, No. 2, 1946) with the permission of the American Physical Therapy Association.

THE SECRETARY OF THE NAVY
WASHINGTON

The Secretary of the Navy takes pleasure in commending

LIEUTENANT SIGNE BRUNNSTROM
UNITED STATES NAVAL RESERVE

for service as set forth in the following

CITATION:

"For outstanding service as Officer-in-Charge of the Physical Therapy Department, United States Naval Hospital, Mare Island, California, from August 1943, to October 1945. Acting as a trained physical therapist and as an instructor in physical therapy, Lieutenant Brunnstrom, by her enthusiasm, stimulated patients to put forth increasingly greater efforts in accelerating their physical rehabilitation. Her skill, sympathetic understanding and determination were of incalculable benefit in the rehabilitation of amputees and other war casualties and her steadfast performance of duty reflects the highest credit upon Lieutenant Brunnstrom and the United States Naval Service."

A copy of this citation has been made a part of Lieutenant Brunnstrom's official record, and she is hereby authorized to wear the Commendation Ribbon.

James Forrestal
Secretary of the Navy

Commendation from James Forrestal, Secretary of the Navy for Signe's work at Mare Island from 1943-45.

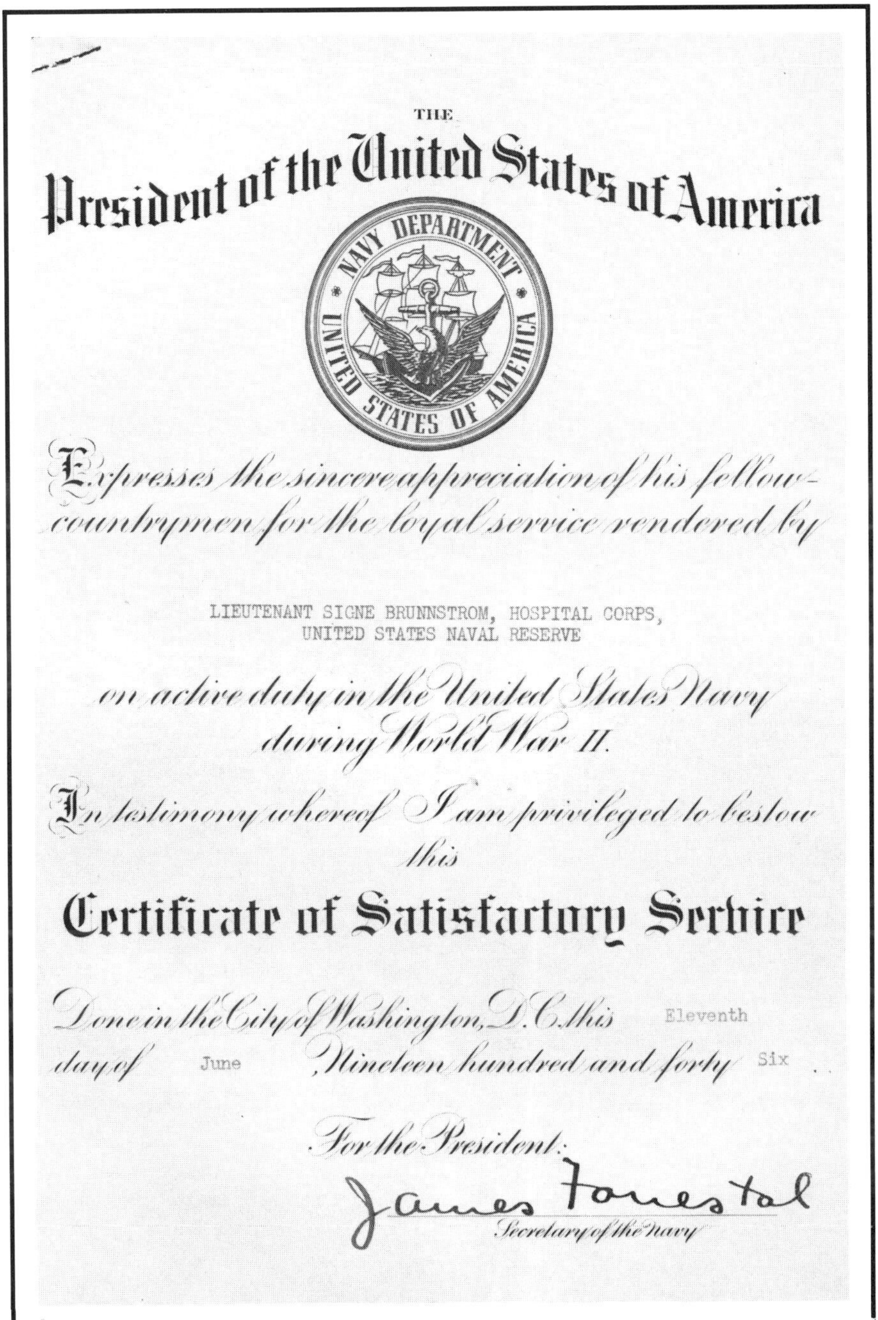

THE

President of the United States of America

Expresses the sincere appreciation of his fellow-countrymen for the loyal service rendered by

LIEUTENANT SIGNE BRUNNSTROM, HOSPITAL CORPS,
UNITED STATES NAVAL RESERVE

on active duty in the United States Navy during World War II.

In testimony whereof I am privileged to bestow this

Certificate of Satisfactory Service

Done in the City of Washington, D.C. this Eleventh day of June, Nineteen hundred and forty Six.

For the President:

James Forrestal

Secretary of the Navy

Certificate of Satisfactory Service from the Secretary of the Navy for Signe's naval service, 1946.

The Physical Therapy Review

Official Publication of The American Physical Therapy Association

Vol. 33 | August 1953 | Number 8

Head Posture and Muscle Tone

Clinical Observations by A. Simons*

Abstracted by Signe Brunnstrom

Introduction

The principles which govern the appearance of tonic neck and labyrinthine reflexes in decerebrate and in intact animals were discovered and reported by Magnus and de Kleijn. An abstract of chapter III of Magnus' book "Körperstellung" appeared in the *Physical Therapy Review*, June 1953.

Observations of the appearance of these reflexes in human beings have been reported in medical literature. Such observations were made on patients with brain lesions which were so severe that practically all cerebral influences were blocked, thus eliminating voluntary control. The patients' conditions, therefore, were very much like that of a decerebrate animal. It was assumed that a severe lesion was necessary in order that "no voluntary impulses disturb the observations" (Magnus). In these severe lesions the reflexes were elicited by passive head motions.

Clinical observations by A. Simons made it clear that extensive brain damage is not a prerequisite for the appearance of neck and labyrinthine reflexes. They can be observed in hemiplegics, although in these cases the reflexes do not appear readily on passive motions. Mild changes in the muscle tone of the affected extremities are likely to occur on passive motions, but cannot always be clearly demonstrated, and a reinforcement of the reflex is needed. Simons reinforced the reflex by having the patient actively contract muscles in other parts of the body. Usually he had the patient squeeze a dynamometer in the unaffected hand, but resisted hip or elbow motions of the unaffected side also were utilized, and sometimes resisted motions of the affected leg to reinforce the reflex in the arm. By this method involuntary motions, called "associated motions," appeared in the affected extremities. It was then demonstrated that the position of the head determined the pattern of the "associated motions," in accordance with the rules for tonic neck and labyrinthine reflexes.

The material contained in the abstract which follows was published, in part, in Zentralbl. f. Neurol. 39:132, 1920, under the title, "Kopfhaltung und Muskeltonus." During the years which followed, the author's observations continued and more clinical data were collected. The article was revised, enlarged, and republished in 1923 under the same title. The following abstract was made from this latter article. (Zeitschr. f. d. ges. Neurol. u. Psycho. 80: 499-549, 1923)

S. Brunnstrom

Study of the influences of the position of the head on the tone† of the extremities is compara-

Consultant, Kessler Institute for Rehabilitation, West Orange, New Jersey; Consultant, Veterans' Administration.

* From the First Medical Clinic of the University of Berlin.

† Tone as used in this article designates an involuntary tension in skeletal muscle.

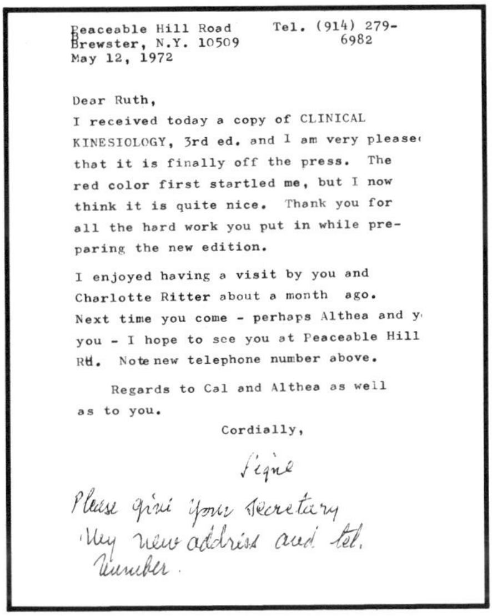

Peaceable Hill Road Tel. (914) 279-6982
Brewster, N.Y. 10509
May 12, 1972

Dear Ruth,

I received today a copy of CLINICAL KINESIOLOGY, 3rd ed. and I am very pleased that it is finally off the press. The red color first startled me, but I now think it is quite nice. Thank you for all the hard work you put in while preparing the new edition.

I enjoyed having a visit by you and Charlotte Ritter about a month ago. Next time you come - perhaps Althea and you - I hope to see you at Peaceable Hill Rd. Note new telephone number above.

Regards to Cal and Althea as well as to you.

Cordially,

Signe

Please give your secretary my new address and tel. number.

Signe's letter to Ruth Dickinson about Ruth's revision of Clinical Kinesiology.

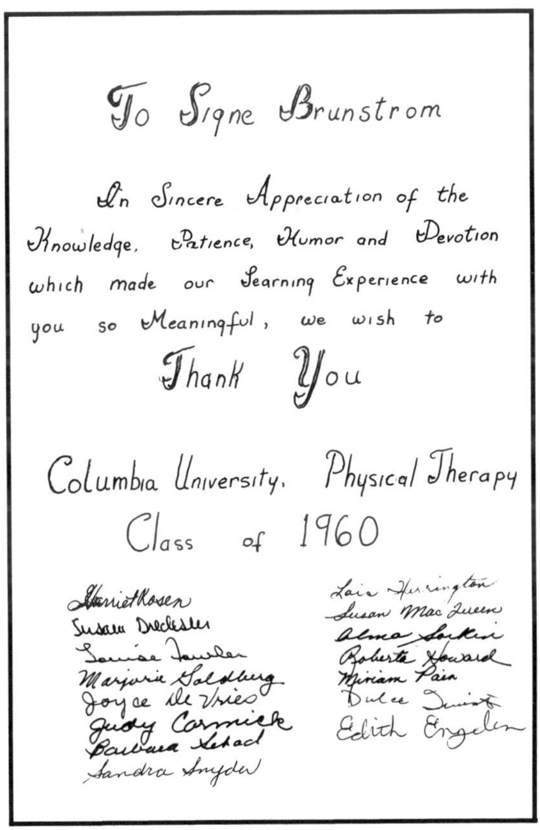

To Signe Brunstrom

In Sincere Appreciation of the Knowledge, Patience, Humor and Devotion which made our Learning Experience with you so Meaningful, we wish to

Thank You

Columbia University, Physical Therapy
Class of 1960

Harriet Rosen
Susan Drechsler
Louise Fowler
Marjorie Goldberg
Joyce De Vries
Judy Cormick
Barbara Sehad
Sandra Snyder

Lois Herrington
Susan MacQueen
Alma Sorkin
Roberta Howard
Miriam Pain
Dulce Smith
Edith Engelen

One of Signe's most cherished possessions.

Chapter Six

No Time For Retirement

During the first three months of 1964 at Stanford University, California, in Palo Alto, Signe taught Kinesiology 220 in the Division of Physical Therapy. She substituted for the ailing Marian Williams, Associate Professor of Physical Therapy. While there, Signe accepted an invitation to give a workshop at Rancho Los Amigos in Downey. She referred to the workshop in a letter written a year later to Mary Eleanor Brown:

> With an admission fee of $10, (which I thought was much too much) and an attendance of 70–80 PTs, OTs, and M.D.s, there was plenty of money left over after they had reimbursed me for traveling expenses from Stanford and given me a fee of $100.

Back in Carmel, New York in late spring, Signe once again picked up her former work and consulting schedule. She also devoted time to preparing another article for submission to the Journal of the American Physical Therapy Association. The article, *Walking Patterns for Adult Patients with Hemiplegia* appeared in the journal almost a year later (Volume 45, No.1).

Added to her activities was the revision of the 1962 edition of *Clinical Kinesiology* in preparation for the second edition. Much of the work was accomplished in late 1964 and carried over throughout 1965. Signe felt a revision was necessary, as she found many areas of omission in the first edition. They may have been minor changes, but being a perfectionist, she intended to see that a new edition would be updated and correct. For example, in the first edition, on page 14, there is a diagram depicting the algebraic summation of vector forces along a common line of action. The line was divided into three parts. Signe wanted to clarify the diagram by adding "A","B", and "C" to designate the three parts. On page 213, referring to patients, there was a word change from "post-poliomyelitis" to "post-poliomyelitic." Page 49 mentions "the epicondyle." Signe decided to add a definition: "epi, upon; kondylos, condyle."

The inside and back covers of Signe's personal copy of the first edition include 38 notations for changes, and many more are scattered throughout the text. On March 11, in Philadelphia, she met with a Miss Anderson of F. A. Davis to discuss the revisions. The manuscript was finalized by the next week, and on March 17 it was sent to the publisher.

In the preface to the second edition, Signe wrote:

> The organization in this second edition of Clinical Kinesiology remains essentially the same as that in the first edition. The new material which has been inserted concerns mainly recent electromyographic studies which significantly add to our knowledge of joint movement and muscle function. A brief report of these studies is given, mainly for the purpose of drawing the reader's attention to these publications which deserve being read in their entirety.

By November 30, Signe had the galleys. The index and bibliography were prepared in December. The project was ready for publication.

Actually, 1965 was a year of many accomplishments, some difficulties and the appearance of a spectre of illness.

Signe never did only one thing at a time. This is best exemplified by following her activities throughout the year.

While working on the revisions for the second edition of *Clinical Kinesiology*, she decided to assume the responsibility for the preparation of a monograph on movement therapy in hemiplegia. Much of the work was based on the manual prepared at the Burke Rehabilitation Foundation. In early January, Helen Hislop called Signe and suggested that she sign a contract with Paul Hoeber of the Hoeber Medical Division of Harper and Row. Signe's diary states, "I did not do so, premature."

Once again, with the assistance of the faculty in the Physical and Occupational Therapy Departments at Columbia, Signe helped develop a grant application which was submitted to the Vocational Rehabilitation Administration on April 19. Mary Callahan, Director of Courses in Physical Therapy was listed as the grant training program director with Robert C. Darling, M.D., as Chairman of the Department of Physical Medicine and Rehabilitation. The training period was listed as September 1, 1965 through August 31, 1966. Signe was listed as a 1/3 part-time instructor at a salary of $2,500 from the grant and $500 from the program's funds. The proposed "training project" was described as follows:

> This application is for financial assistance for the preparation of a manual on the subject MOVEMENT THERAPY FOR STROKE PATIENTS. The manual will deal with specific techniques of movement and with the rationale for such techniques, based on clinical observation of the motor behavior of these patients and as much as possible on scientific material in the field of neurophysiology and neuropatholgy. (Magnus, Simons, Twitchell, etc.)

Mary Callahan also wrote about the "considerable experience" Signe had in the management of stroke patients, as well as being considered "one of the outstanding specialists in the understanding of human motion." The total amount of funds requested for the "teaching grant" or production of the manual was

$4,247. Included in the application was a request for funding of 20 traineeships amounting to $50,000. In all the grant request was for $54,247. The grant was approved on August 6.

One can now look back and wonder what would have happened to Signe's two major publications if the drive for funds had not been spearheaded by the directors and faculty at Columbia. Ruth Dickinson wrote in 1986, "It's a source of pride for Columbia University's Program in Physical Therapy that with Mary Callahan's expert leadership we secured grant funds to help Signe publish two texts that have become such classics in our field. Scores of students and therapists have benefited from these writings and Signe's influence continues for future therapists who will read literature based on her teachings."

By September 20, Signe was setting up statistical data for the project. She intended to use material from patients seen at the Neurological Institute in 1961 and 1962. Assisting her with the patient records was Althea Jones, then an instructor and member of the faculty. Althea's responsibility was to assist Signe with her teaching and help gather data on the evaluation of the hemiplegic patient. Throughout September and October, Althea and Signe prepared test forms and did case histories on patients at the Neurological Institute and at Burke. According to Althea, "Signe insisted on developing a reliable, valid instrument with which to measure the patient's movement characteristics before including in her book her thoughts on the recovery stages of the hemiplegic patient." Althea quickly recognized that Signe "set high standards for herself and instilled this value in all who associated with her. She was a very disciplined professional and has always been committed to accuracy in reporting."

Althea recalled a very special event that illustrated Signe's dedication to research and her disciplined nature. In mid-February, Althea spent the day at Bullet Hole Road compiling findings of the assessment of patients. Did the patients recover in a certain sequence (Stage I, II, etc.)?

Papers were spread around the room. It was a cold day but the room was heated by a round kerosene stove. Signe's excitement was showing as the data fell into place, as she had hypothesized. I was typing some of the records and my fingers were losing their flexibility because of the cold. Imagine my surprise when Signe said, "I can't stand a hot room" and proceeded to remove the small stove. I must say I too began to get caught up in the excitement of the findings and I forgot about the cold. Her enthusiasm was contagious and this enthusiasm always existed when working with Signe. I feel honored to have had a close educational experience with her. Much of her wisdom came from her close observations of movement and questioning why these movements occurred. As a mentor Signe taught me "The doors of Wisdom are never shut."

This was only the beginning of a great amount of work that would be required before the new text would be published. In its final form, it would not be a monograph but one of the most important publications devoted to treatment approaches for the hemiplegic patient, and it would be Signe Brunnstrom's third published book.

Another major activity that required a lot of time in 1965 came as a result of a phone call from Mary Eleanor Brown of Cleveland on January 25. She invited Signe to participate in a continuing education program planned for October at Case Western Reserve University (CWRU). Mary Eleanor explained, "It was one of thirty continuing education courses offered by the Graduate Physical Therapy Curriculum under the direction of Geneva R. Johnson." During the phone conversation, Mary Eleanor detected that Signe was not her usual self: "My concerns over Signe's well-being stem from this time as she expressed fears of neurophysiologic symptoms. She was under great stress regarding her living quarters." Regardless of whatever was developing, Signe agreed to participate.

The program was to include three different units under the general title of "Human Motion: Review and Application of Neurophysiologic Principles with Emphasis on Hemiplegia." It was scheduled for October 14 through 20. The first unit, primarily dealing with a review of neuroanatomy and neurophysiology, would be open to all health professions personnel. Tuition cost was $25. The lecturers would be Norman Taslitz, Ph.D., Assistant Professor of Physical Therapy and Instructor in the Department of Anatomy of the School of Medicine at CWRU, and Don Lehmkuhl, Ph.D., Assistant Professor of Physical Therapy and Senior Instructor in Physiology in CRWU's Department of Physiology in the School of Medicine.

Signe was to participate in "Unit Two", which would only be open to physical therapists (graduates of approved physical therapy schools). Only 15 persons would be registered because of the required supervised clinical instruction. The cost for the 10-day workshop was $150, and included attendance at the other two units as well as supplies and materials.

The plan also included Signe offering a one-day session on Saturday, October 23, open to all health professional personnel. This session would cover the application of neurophysiological principles to training procedures for hemiplegic patients. The lecture demonstrations were to include participation by those physical therapists from "Unit Two". The cost of the one-day session was $10.

Mary Eleanor followed up the invitation in a letter of February 25th with more details. Signe responded in a letter of March 3:

> I would like to spend as much time as possible in the hospitals. Lectures are all right (and needed), but techniques can only be learned in the clinic. On the days that lectures are scheduled in the evening, I should be able to work in the hospitals in the morning, the other days mornings and afternoons, unless it proves too fatiguing.

During the next several months, Signe planned her part of the program and looked forward to being in Cleveland in October.

Unfortunately, she was troubled by a major problem relating to her property on Bullet Hole Road. Even though she was aware as far back as 1955 that someday the State of New York was planning to build a major highway through Putnam County, she did not think it would disturb her land. On January 4, 1965 her notes indicate, "highway crew to set off dynamite charges to determine depth of rocks on my property." All the peace and tranquility of the rolling hills was to be shattered with road construction. Signe's house and four acres of land would be appropriated by the State and taken over for the highway. Knowing how much Signe loved her home and land, the news must have been devastating. Problems with the state and highway authorities occupied her mind for several years. There would be many meetings with state representatives, legal people and friends. Signe could not fight the system. Referring to the worrisome litigation, Mary Eleanor Brown said the major reason Signe could not possibly oppose the situation was that "she was not a combative person in any sense." All Signe could do was raise questions, seek some answers and continue with her professional work.

Signe took a plane to Cleveland on June 30, where she was a participant in the APTA Annual Conference held at the Sheraton Cleveland Hotel. (The cost of her room was $8.50 a night.) She lectured and demonstrated on two hemiplegic patients. While at the conference, one of the brightest moments in 1965 (and in her professional life,) came when Signe was recognized for her research in physical therapy. On July 1, the master physical therapist, Signe Brunnstrom, was presented with the first Marian Williams Award. The presentation was made at APTA's annual banquet by Mary Elizabeth Kolb, Association President. While it was an occasion of great honor, Signe initially had an adverse reaction. Fran Tappan, standing nearby, described Signe as "pale and sweating." Signe told Fran she was not sure she could go through with the acceptance of the award, as she felt "as if she was having a stroke." The presentation did take place without any problems, and photographs were taken, followed by a reception. The APTA's action in recognizing Signe was well-founded.

The news release prepared on the event stated: "Miss Brunnstrom is recognized throughout the medical community for her contributions to locomotion and exercise, particularly for patients with strokes. Amputee patients all over the world are beneficiaries of the work she has done in developing training methods for the use of artificial limbs." Ms. Kolb presented Signe with a large bronze plaque and a citation. The citation read:

WHEREAS: The American Physical Therapy Association has established the Marian Williams Award for research that has been conceived, conducted and reported by a physical therapist, and

WHEREAS: Throughout your professional career you have exhibited the high standards of performance in research worthy of this award, and

WHEREAS: You have faithfully reported your careful observations in professional journals and reference books so that they are shared by all of your colleagues, and

WHEREAS: Your particular interests in kinesiology and human locomotion have led to notable advances in patient care, be, it, therefore,

RESOLVED: That this tribute of the Association be presented to you, Signe Brunnstrom, for fundamental and significant contributions to the development of the profession of physical therapy through research.

The citation was signed by Mary Elizabeth Kolb, President, and Dorothy I. Briggs, Chairman of the Editorial Board. (The large plaque was held by Signe for many years and then passed on to Ruth Dickinson of Columbia University. She later presented it to the Archives of Physical Therapy in the APTA office in Alexandria, Virginia.

Don Lehmkuhl, of CWRU was at the annual conference. It was an opportunity for him to meet Signe and discuss the forthcoming October workshop. Since he was to be responsible for a major part of the workshop, he arranged to talk with Signe after a conference session, about 5 P.M. Norman Taslitz, also a presenter for the October program, accompanied him. Don described the meeting in a letter of August 16, 1985:

> Signe appeared extremely pleased to meet with us. Her eyes sparkled with enthusiasm as we described the features of the graduate physical therapy educational program at CRWU. She was full of questions about the design of the curriculum, how we integrated the basic sciences, clinical sciences and clinical practice, and how we guided each of the students in planning and conducting a research project. Then we began discussing our understanding of the possible physiological mechanisms that may influence the recovery of motor control in patients with neurological disorders. To substantiate a particular point, she would dig through a suitcase of reprints, letters and notebooks until she found the document needed. About midnight we realized that we hadn't eaten dinner, so we adjourned to a nearby sandwich shop. At 2 A.M., we decided to stop picking at each other's brain and get some rest. She had to leave the next day, so I didn't see her again until she returned for the workshop.

The Continuing Education Program at CWRU went off on schedule. Sixteen physical therapists were signed up for the full course. Don Lehmkuhl recently wrote:

> I can honestly say that the opportunity to teach a short course with Signe was one of the highlights of my career. Her powers of observation were phenomenal and her depth and breadth of knowledge were extensive. But she never behaved in a "superior-than-thou"

manner. Her interpersonal relationships with patients and other professionals were kind, gracious and humanistic.

Arthur Spell, P.T., from the Veterans Administration Hospital in Coatesville, Pennsylvania, was among the select group in the full course. Presently at the Laurel Road Physical Therapy Center in Stratford, New Jersey, he wrote on June 20, 1985:

> Signe as I remember was a very dynamic person who was extremely knowledgeable and serious about her techniques yet aware and appreciative of the other various methods of treatment. She demonstrated a sense of humor yet maintaining her serious professionalism. It was indeed my expressed privilege, pleasure and reward of having the experience of studying under and working with Signe. Her presence, patience and contributions will long be of value and remembered.

Another therapist in the full course was Floyd Spurgeon of Alliance, Ohio. He wrote (May 20, 1985):

> I think the most lasting impression Signe made on me was the use of her hands. She had such a touch, strong yet gentle, firm yet kind that patients seemed to respond to her direction before they realized what they were doing. I never heard a patient say to her "I can't do that" as she had such a positive approach they didn't have a chance to object. Her calmness and delightful accent made one listen carefully and react positively to all she asked. Signe had the ability and a certain humbleness to transmit her knowledge in such a way that her students were made to feel as capable as she.
>
> The course under her teaching provided me with a confidence and ability to treat many patients through the years with many recoveries that otherwise could have been failures . . . I have only one regret and that is that I did not let her know of my respect, admiration

and yes, love of her, and how much I have used her techniques to help others over the years.

Major Mary J. Torp, (now retired and living in Del City, Oklahoma,) a physical therapist with the Army, attached to Walter Reed Hospital in Washington, D.C., also attended the course. She made a major contribution to the program by taking copious notes. Major Torp recalled (February 26, 1985):

> I went to all the hospitals and clinics and observed the others' clinical instructions, taking extensive notes. I turned these into a sort of text, which I sent to Miss B., to correct and review, and then had it mimeographed for my classmates. While in Cleveland, Signe was living on the grant she received to prepare the book on hemiplegia. We were all helping her by picking out what we thought was valuable. I thought I was helping by putting together some of her classroom and clinic notes, sayings and doing what possibly helped her to organize her material, but I doubt it. I think she had it all set up before she came to Cleveland and was just leaving out material she found irrelevant at that point. Or at least leaving out things which could be eliminated from most evaluations, in order to save space, and allow for improvement in a later edition.

Mary Torp also became aware of Signe's personal problems as they talked during evening walks in a park with a small lake near the hotel:

> Signe was trying to save money as she had no income so she did not eat out, staying in her room and studying each night, eating provisions she had brought with her. She said she had always answered the call for knowledge and sought answers, and suddenly found she had not enough social security retirement credits, no college teachers retirement, no means of support except her royalties from her books. She was considering at one time going back to Sweden as she thought she would be eligible for a retirement income there.

> She also was worried and expressed concern for her home and the old barn being destroyed by the freeway coming through, and not wanting her "Bullet Hole" changed. She liked the location as she could get into New York City to do research and loved the name of the road.
>
> Although Signe thought her teaching at the course was hasty and sketchy, her discussions in class and clinic were a marvel to me, even though I had seen some of the best in action, both physicians and physical therapists. I rate her tops in being able to tell "why" as well as "what." Part of her value to our profession was her inquisitive mind, but part was her willingness to make the sacrifice to do research, knowing how important it was that it be done. She knew that her language gift was intended for more hard work, digging out answers in the various languages she knew (and learned just to be able to find more answers).

An important observation was made by Mary Torp when she noted how ill Signe had become during the course:

> She was having severe physical problems, coughing up blood (but not letting anyone know. I saw it during a break or two and she just shrugged it off and kept going) and having to walk very fast around the park after her day was over, getting blood back up to her brain. I think she always took a nap first. I know she had to turn in early as I would get materials from her to copy each evening and had to return them prior to 9 P.M.

Geneva Johnson, former Director of the PT program at Western Reserve contributed her comments about Signe in a letter of January 5, 1986:

> Miss Brunnstrom had a mesmerizing quality about her when she worked with a patient who had a cerebral vascular accident. She would greet a patient she had never seen before and within minutes that person had responded by performing a movement she requested. The patient and the audience were equally astonished at

her ability to elicit such a rapid response. She worked her magic under the glare of bright lights, on a stage in a crowded room, with patients who were strangers to her. But, she and the patient were oblivious to their surroundings as she talked, soothed, and directed the patient. Energy, positive expectations, and genuine caring flowed into the patient through her marvelous hands.

When I speak of Miss Brunnstrom, the words are accompanied by movements of my hands. Those movements seem essential in describing her and occur automatically. I visualize her hands moving gracefully, gently, and purposefully—reaching toward the patient. Then I remember a smile of pure pleasure on the face of the delighted patient as he watched his hand open and close under her direction. I also remember the merriment in her eyes and the soft laughter as she exchanged comments with patients and colleagues as she worked or lectured.

Another physical therapist in the workshop was Betty Canan (now of the University of Alabama at Birmingham, Allied Health Department). In a letter of January 20, 1986, she wrote:

Patients never forgot Miss Brunnstrom. She radiated warmth, compassion, and understanding. The patient's walk of life or level of intelligence mattered not one iota in her behavior toward that individual as a human being. Again, I recall her immediate rapport with Archie, who never failed to ask about her whenever he saw one of our P.T.'s. Archie served as a demonstration patient during one of Miss Brunnstrom's workshops. A forty year old man with many limitations, I shall never forget the look of pride on his face when he presented Miss Brunnstrom a wallet he had made and wanted to give her as a token of his appreciation. Her reaction (and you know she must have received hundreds of such gifts) was just beautiful—like a kid receiving his first puppy.

> Signe's warm sense of humor was another delightful attribute. I can remember the twinkle in her eye when she joked about Mary Eleanor Brown's attempt to get her organized for this workshop, covering every little detail—and Mary Eleanor, with a twinkle in her own eyes, just kept on trying!

During the workshop, Mary Eleanor Brown had Signe moving "at quite a clip" in the two week period. "All of the participants," according to Geneva Johnson, "wanted to spend time alone with Signe. Everyone had that opportunity in a clinical setting. The course was a wonderful success."

After Cleveland, Signe relaxed for a very brief time. She continued to meet with the staff at the Burke Rehabilitation Center and worked on her research. By the end of November she had completed the outline for a spring course on the application of neurophysiologic principles to human motion to be offered at Columbia University. Proofreading of the revised *Clinical Kinesiology* text also took a lot of time.

Ending the year, on December 12, Signe's diary indicated "worked on a paper for the APTA Journal."

New Year's Day, 1966, was Signe's 68th birthday.

The new year found Signe deeply involved in the preparation of the hemiplegia manual. Her investigative studies continued at Burke and the Neurological Institute. She also arranged for the photographic services of a Mr. Crew of Crew Studios in Carmel, N.Y. to take professional photographs of her patient demonstrations at Burke. Since the work on the manual was supported by a VRA grant, she employed a Mrs. Bird to do some of the typing of the manuscript. In addition, she arranged with an artist, Phillip Carson of Uniondale, N.Y., to prepare drawings and illustrations. Signe's schedule called for testing of patients, preparation of illustrations, directing photography, researching case histories and completing rough drafts—all while working with patients and staff at Burke.

"Lou" Loescher was a PT on the staff at the time. Now Coordinator of Rehab Services at St. Luke's Hospital of Kansas City, she wrote on October 19, 1984:

Ms. Brunnstrom was completing her book on hemiplegia. She worked very closely with a couple of my patients and I am embarrassed to admit to it, but my picture is in the book on more than one page.

This past week I had the pleasure of teaching the "Brunnstrom Techniques" to the University of Kansas students. It brought back fond memories of a very dynamic, caring person. The one thing that I feel should be emphasized about her technique is her basic belief that the "sensory input effects the motor output." Ms. Brunnstrom so lived that principle in her treatment of patients through body language, voice commands, and manual stimulation techniques. There was and still is no doubt in my mind that above all else the verbal commands and her dynamic enthusiastic attitude made the difference in the patient's functional outcomes.

The staff at Burke at that time was most fortunate to have learned the technique from her, but more important we learned an approach to the patient . . . remembering the "lady" gives me goose bumps, blurry eyes and makes me proud to be a physical therapist, maybe that says it all.

In April, Signe again traveled to 630 West 168th Street in Upper Manhattan when she started lecturing in Kinesiology 206 in the Columbia PT program. The course consisted of 12 two-hour lectures to 46 students. As always, students were considered very important. The planning of course material and presentations was a priority as Signe gave all she had to those she taught.

For two days in April, the twenty-second and twenty third, Signe was at the Harmarville Rehabilitation Center in Pittsburgh, giving a continuing education course on neurological approaches to the hemiplegic. Arrangements were made by James Herrington, P.T., one of the participants in the workshop at CWRU. Jim wrote, "My very pleasant experience in 1965, at the Western Reserve workshop and the needs of my staff were the basis for planning this seminar." As the Director of

Physical Therapy at Harmarville, he felt the need to develop a more dynamic program in the treatment of stroke patients as explained in his letter of December 29, 1985:

> Signe, through her understanding of the neuromuscular deficits and methods necessary to meet the needs of stroke patients in evaluation and treatment, was the only physical therapist who could present what I thought was current and effective. She was very well accepted. There were 200 participants which included 20 physicians of neurological, orthopedic and psychiatric specialties. Also attending were Lucy Blair, then the executive director of APTA, Mary Elizabeth Kolb, APTA President and representatives from insurance companies and other third party payers. Signe dealt with all aspects of neurological needs through her presentations utilizing patients. She reproduced a very extensive bibliography. She demonstrated synergistic patterns which are still being used by PTs who take the time to treat stroke patients.

Jim also wrote about his introduction of Signe at Harmarville. ''Signe,'' he said, ''commented that she was not used to speaking to physicians about the care of the stroke patient, since stroke patients were the step-children of medicine, at least as they, the physicians saw them.'' Jim felt that Signe ''was a strong person and had great conviction about her knowledge and what she presented and was very seldom challenged because we all knew she was so well prepared.''

Signe saw more results of her writing and research when she had another article, *Motor Testing Procedures in Hemiplegia: Based on Sequential Recovery Stages*, published in the Journal of the American Physical Therapy Association, (1966, 46:357- 374).

July 26 was a bitter day for Signe. She met with Karl Beers of Poughkeepsie, the right-of-way agent for the new highway, who stated that, ''road construction would begin in late fall or early winter.'' Signe found that difficult to believe, but accepted the fact, and in anticipation of the destruction of her cottage (the coop), planned to move to the basement of her ‘‘Hill House’’. She gave notice to her tenant, but it would be months before she could move in. Her sister, Elsa, arrived from Sweden on September 20 to help with the move. A few pieces of furniture, four oak chairs, two other chairs and an oak chest were prepared for shipment to Ingegerd. It cost $128.50 to ship it all to Sweden. Out of discussions with Elsa, consideration was given to moving part of the cottage to the acreage that would remain after the state appropriated what was needed for the highway. Signe intended to look into that possibility. Elsa returned to Sweden on October 10, and Signe was left once again to handle all the problems.

Aside from packing, having Thanksgiving with some friends, lecturing at Burke Rehab, visiting the Castle Point Veterans Administration Hospital and working on the hemiplegia manual, Signe received an invitation to speak at the Annual Conference of the American Academy for Cerebral Palsy planned for December 3–6 at the Roosevelt Hotel in New Orleans. There was to be a panel of ‘‘experts’’ who proposed various treatment approaches for neurological conditions. It may have sounded too controversial for Signe, or she could not give the time and energy to such an undertaking. She did not accept the invitation.

Joan Mohr, P.T. of Cresskill, New Jersey, remembers that Academy meeting very well. ‘‘ ‘It was quite a session.’ Ms. Mohr indicated there were presentations by Margaret Knott, Margaret Rood, Berte Bobath, and Robert Doman. ‘‘After all the presentations were given, they were torn apart by the physicians who really were hitting at Doman. The presenters each were asked if they had anything to say. No one said much except Mrs. Bobath. Her comment was direct and to the point. ‘If all medical professions feel that way about all presenters, we might as well go home.’ She was the only one who stood up to the physicians and was respected for the rest of her comments as well.’’

It is very likely that, had Signe Brunnstrom been present, she would have totally agreed with Mrs. Bobath.

Lectures and clinical work continued at the Burke Center. Thanks to the cooperation of Tony DeRosa, Signe was able to obtain her additional 150 copies of the hemiplegia manual used by the students. She personally picked up the multilithed materials on December 22 and delivered them to the Columbia PT program.

Signe's year ended once again thinking of other people. She had a request from Ruby Decker of Galveston, Texas, who organized a School of Physiotherapy at the West Pakistan Society for the Rehabilitation of the Disabled in Lahore. Ruby designed the curriculum on the basis of what was taught at the PT school of the University of Texas Medical Branch in Galveston. Included in therapeutic exercise was Signe Brunnstrom's program for brain- damaged patients, particularly those resulting in spasticity and athetosis. Ruby wrote on December 10, 1984: "Signe's approach was scientific and her methods practical. She kindly responded to my requests for literature about her methods, which was placed in the clinical library at the school." On December 27, 1966, Signe's diary indicated, "packed books for West Pakistan and Ruby Decker."

New Year's Day, 1967, was Signe's 69th birthday. There was no time for celebration. She started the year with much on her mind. Problems related to the highway took much of her time and interfered with her work schedule. Typical of a major public construction project, the work on Highway 84 did not begin on time. The family in the Hill House still did not vacate. It was a difficult time.

In spite of all the distractions, the hemiplegia manual was completed. On January 11, Mary Callahan sent five copies of the publication to V.R.A. Division of Training Chief Cecile Hillyer. Mary indicated a total of 150 copies had been prepared, "and would be made available to both students of Occupational Therapy and Physical Therapy at Columbia University that Spring and for the academic year 1967-68 for use in courses in kinesiology, clinical applications and therapeutic exercise." She also mentioned that Signe would continue to work on the manual and solicit criticism, and "eventually the publication might be available to all interested professional purposes." In Miss Hillyer's acknowledgment of receiving the manuals, she wrote January 18, "It was our pleasure to share in the cost of developing this fine teaching manual, which I know will be a welcome addition to the physical therapy educational programs and graduate therapists.''

Signe was also determined to see the manual in the hands of all therapists. To this end, in early January, she carried the manuscript and many photos, and traveled to New York City to meet with a Mr. Frankenfield at Harper and Row, Publishers. She also recognized that there would be additional work required on the manual and somehow she would have to find time to do it all. She also continued teaching Kinesiology 108 in the Columbia PT program, which was shared with Althea Jones. By the end of January, Signe's lecture series at Burke was completed. This gave her some additional time to devote to enlarging the manual. One of the first steps was to arrange for the selection of patients to be used in photographs for the publication.

Another honor came to Signe on February 16, when she was invited to give the prestigious Mary McMillian lecture at the September 8 annual conference of the APTA. Once again, Signe was unable to undertake such a responsibility and did not accept the invitation.

In late February, Signe arranged to offer three instructional days at Goldwater Memorial Hospital in New York City. She held two sessions as planned, but the third was canceled and later rescheduled. The change was necessitated by her concern for working on the hemiplegia book.

The contract, or agreement to produce, the hemiplegic manuscript for Harper and Row was signed by Signe on February 11 and by the publisher on February 25. It called for the author to deliver the manuscript in one year. (That became an unrealistic date for Signe as the months went by.)

On March 19, she met with Dr. Meda and Yasuko Fukuya of the Central Rehabilitation Service of the University of Tokyo Hospital. They toured the Neurological Institute and were most impressed with Signe's ideas on rehabilitation of hemiplegic patients. Referring to this visit, Signe wrote, ''my day with the Japanese doctor, a neurologist, and his physical therapist was very interesting and rewarding.''

A bright spot appeared in Signe's notes in mid-March. She wrote, "some of my professional friends in Cleveland are working toward having me be honored by the Western Reserve University with an honorary doctor's degree for my professional achievements." Mary Eleanor Brown wrote, (January 1, 1986,) "I do remember that an honorary degree was proposed at a staff meeting of the Graduate Physical Therapy Curriculum at Case Western Reserve University. I think I made the suggestion but it doesn't really matter whose idea it was." Referring to what transpired after the nomination was made, Geneva Johnson recalled (February 20, 1986): "Signe was not selected to that honor by the Board of Trustees. I do not know how far the nomination went but suspect that she was eliminated from consideration at the level of the President." Signe would have appreciated the honor but her notes indicate she had doubts that it would come to pass. In her own humble way, she wrote, "This I doubt they will succeed in, but even the fact they think I deserve it is encouraging."

The only real travel Signe undertook in the spring was to Detroit March 26–28, where she served as a consultant to "a very interesting clinical research project supported by the Vocational Rehabilitation Administration." The arrangements were made at Mary Taylor's request.

It appeared that Signe really did not want to leave Bullet Hole for any length of time. Not only was she concerned about her two dogs and the potential construction of the highway, but she had to handle many business matters. Another meeting with the right-of-way agent on March 11 proved more frustrating. The state had established a "claim", following their assessment of the property to be taken. It consisted of a lump sum of $15,000. In a letter of March 16, 1967, to her sister Ingegerd, Signe indicated that the amount of money offered by the state was supposed to be compensation for three acres of pasture and woodland, one acre of landscaped ground, proximity damage to Hill House (loss of selling value,) proximity damage to the spring House and spring and a new septic field by Hill House. She had conservatively estimated the value at $19,500 after she had two real estate business people give an even higher estimate. The estimate Signe offered did not include the four-room cottage and garage, and the "barn, 200 years old with hand-hewn beams, pegs and square nails." Signe, in desperation, looked into what a cottage of the same size would cost and it came to approximately $22,650, without the building of retaining walls and a driveway.

What the state did not typically recognize was all the personal work Signe had done on her land and how impossible it would be to replace any of the many trees and bushes she planted. Among the items mentioned in the letter to Ingegerd were:

> Down at the cottage I have one huge Lindentree (my pride and joy) four ordinary spruces, one silver spruce, eight other evergreens, a large apple tree, a Bartlett pear tree, a plum tree, a vegetable garden, beautiful lawns, a slope full of narcissus, two privet hedges, two forsythia hedges, an 18 inch deep constructed driveway and all kinds of flowering bushes, including eight mountain laurels. Duplicating all this is impossible, even if I spent a fortune on it.

Signe went to a real estate agent and put the Hill House up for sale for $20,000. She was told she could get about $18,000 and that she "would be lucky to sell it all." As part of the sale, she would have to give up more acreage. The highway would still curve around the house and be seen from three sides.

An interesting option was made available to Signe. She could buy back the cottage and barn from the state for "salvage value", at a minimal cost of $75 for the house and $25 for the barn. She explained her dilemma:

> If I buy back the cottage and barn, I will have to flatten everything with the ground. It would be quite possible to move part of the cottage at a reasonable price by a company from Danbury. They would do it for $1,000 and put it on poles over over an excavated area so that a foundation could be built under it. It

> would be worthwhile for a builder to do it if he had a place it could be put. I have ground of about ½ an acre where it could be put, but it would be almost like starting from scratch if I were to do it myself and would require so much of my time that I would have no time for professional obligations. Besides, if I cannot sell the Hill House swiftly, I would be stuck with two houses, quite a responsibility financially because of taxes, insurances, maintenance, etc. Also, I am not allowed to buy back a part of the cottage (the new part), it is an all-or-nothing proposition and I still would have the responsibility of demolishing the entire building, which would be quite expensive.

In order to save the 200-year-old barn, Signe made a magnanimous offer to the Historical Society of Putnam County. She believed it then would be preserved. Representatives of the Society regretted they did not have the money to take the barn down and move the valuable parts. ''I offered the barn to them as a gift, but it would be an expensive gift,'' Signe noted.

Snow fell for two days in a raging storm that kept Signe from going to the city. Living in the basement of the Hill House, she passed the time by ''sitting at my desk for a couple of hours, then go out shoveling snow for an hour, the whole thing being repeated over and over again.'' Sixteen to 18 inches of snow fell. Signe received no help from her tenants upstairs. The woman is described by Signe as being ''in her twenties, strong like a bear . . . and her husband keeps his car down the road so he can get out without cleaning the driveway.'' Margit Aden, her long-time friend, did try to help by offering some advice, but as is often the case, Signe stated, ''advice is not much value.'' Margit suggested Signe should write her Congressman from the district and complain about the treatment she received. According to Signe, ''another adviser tells me to write Governor Rockefeller, and a third one tells me that my letter should go directly to the President or Vice-President of the United States! Neither of these advisers suggestions I will follow, for obvious reasons." Since everyone agreed that she was getting a "lousy deal" if she accepted the state's offer, Signe wrote the Department of Public Works to appeal their decision. "It was a last effort, which I am sure will be to no avail, according to the regulations which I have obtained." Signe was a lonely 69-year-old woman in trouble and no one was readily available to offer any real assistance.

Although she set a price for the Hill House, it was necessary to arrange to have a septic field in place before it could be sold. Again, it meant several calls and letters to the inspector from the town of Patterson to come look over the situation. It was three weeks before he came. Signe was told she would have to use a licensed engineer and find a company that would prepare the septic field. She recognized the fact that someone could be interested in the house, "but you can't expect them to buy before the septic field is in order." She also was very unhappy that the Department of Public Works shoved the responsibility on her without giving any information on how much was set aside to pay her for the relocation. She wrote, "They don't seem to care a bit about it and they have already twice refused to give me a detailed account of the assessment."

Signe's plan was to hopefully sell the house, but first she had to have the septic field completed and the "taking line staked out." The line involved her hiring a private surveyor at a cost of $360 because the State engineers or surveyors would not do it. She was aware that the bank would not approve anyone mortgage without a survey. There was no alternative but to have it done.

If the house was sold, Signe intended to look for a place to rent, at least temporarily, until she could build a small place on the remaining triangle acreage she owned. Her other possibility was: "If I can't sell the house within a few months, I will consider staying until the road is finished, at which time it may be easier to sell. But it won't be easy to put up with the bulldozers, the blasting, the dust, etc."

With all the paper work from the state, Signe now had long files from five different sections of the Department of

Public Works, "and often conflicting statements from the various departments."

In early April, things began to fall into place. On the 15th, the tenants living above Signe finally vacated, "at 12 midnight after a noisy party." This now gave her time to clean and paint the area, which actually turned out to be "four months of hard labor. Prospective buyers for the house were "coming and going for several weeks." During this time, Signe "cleaned and refinished the upper floors," while she lived in the basement. Throughout the period involved with the state, faced with all kinds of problems and worries, Signe showed a most unusual strength of character. She was determined to make her way and did not neglect any of her work on the hemiplegic book. She also continued her kinesiology lectures. On May 5 and 6, she went to Minneapolis / St. Paul to conduct a lecture demonstration on treatment of the hemiplegic patients.

The state representatives brought legal papers for her signature on May 17. She was to receive 75 percent of the $15,000. Signing the papers would not influence any future claim. The time was drawing near for the state to take over the cottage and barn. With a very heavy heart Signe, walked around the area on June 4 taking snapshots of all of the familiar places that she had loved for so many years. She also arranged for a bulldozer to remove a large boulder from the triangle where she would eventually build another house.

Signe's notes indicated that on "June 28, 1967, New York State took possession of the cottage, barn and four acres of land. Continued work on manuscript, arranged photos."

One month later, Signe received an offer of $20,000 for the Hill House and one acre of land from Charles Verderese. Of this, $1,200 would go to the real estate man for commission, and "about $18,000 for me." Signe agreed to the sale and the closing was set for August 28. Mr. Verderese recalled his impressions of Signe in a letter of January 27, 1986:

> She was extremely possessive and proud of the house and property. She did a tremendous amount of building

and landscaping herself. She was a very strong and physical woman. She'd think nothing of throwing boulders into a wheelbarrow and hauling them to where she was building a stone fireplace in her new home. She also protected her privacy. I don't recall there being too many people in her life while she was living in her last house. She lived quietly with her two old dogs that she was devoted to. She made regular trips into town to conduct business. She was extremely methodical in her record keeping, as you no doubt have discovered, right down to the last detail. Unfortunately, she found she could not cope with the physical changes having taken place on what was once apple orchards and serenity to her. Signe also had a request from Anthony Ackerman, D.V.M., in September, to purchase a part of an acre (0.824). Signe agreed to that purchase for $350, plus $120 for the survey and deed. In a letter of February 9, 1986, Dr. Ackerman mentioned, "our acquaintance was just that of good neighbors." When he first knew Signe, Dr. Ackerman saw her as "an exceptionally hardworking woman of the old school willing to perform all tasks about her property, with a strength exceptional to a woman and exceptional to her age as well." He wrote: "her character was to my observations tuned to a somewhat higher level than the average of this or any generation. Her standards of honesty were rigid and she expected the same of others. My awareness of her academic accomplishments were sparked by a student in physical therapy who when I mentioned the name of Signe Brunnstrom, reacted as though I had claimed Elvis Presley as a neighbor." Referring to the loss of her home, Dr. Ackerman stated:

I am sure the events relative to this matter had distinct effects on her well-being. The loss of her quiet isolation, the dislocation until she could construct a new home, the disposal of her large house and property, disputes with the state and contamination of her well as a result of the road construction are but a few of the disruptions she experienced. The subsequent, constant roar from I-84 was an unacceptable contrast to the pastoral setting of her former abode.

In late September, Signe looked for a place to rent or buy. (She also turned down a speaking engagement in Buffalo arranged by Barbara Stevenson.) By August 28, she was ready to move to an old farmhouse about three miles from Bullet Hole Rd. She described it as: "a charming old house with a big fireplace. It is quite isolated on a narrow dirt road, which however is a town road, so that it is plowed in winter time." Signe was pleased that the dogs could run free.

Another note in her diary indicated that the move did not stop Signe from her work, " . . . kept working on manuscript for book all month of September." In addition, she called for a new typewriter (cost $95). During October, "completed typing Chapter One, forty-four pages without illustrations." In November, Signe turned down an invitation from Phyllis Lyford for a February, 1968, speaking engagement in Philadelphia.

The deer season began in late November in Putnam County and Signe saw many hunters in the area. She also completed Chapters Two and Three. Although she liked the location of her temporary home, Signe had many problems with the farmhouse. The kitchen became flooded after a rainstorm; the radiator leaked in the living room; the lights went out on November 15; the kersosene stove was inadequate the temperature went to "10 below"; and the road was always slippery with ice and snow. Signe decided to move, and found an apartment in Putnam Terrace which would be available on January 1. It didn't come too soon since on December 25, in the old farmhouse, Signe noted, "water pipes to toilet frozen over." It took Signe three days to prepare for moving. On December 31 she packed a carload of items and, with a hired man and truck, drove to the new apartment. A snowstorm did not make the job easy. The second load was moved on January 1. Happy 70th Birthday, Signe B!

Chapter Seven

Brief Encounters

From her rented apartment, Signe continued typing the hemiplegia manuscript during most of January, 1968. This led to another conference in the city with Mr. Frankenfield of Harper & Row. One week later, Signe saw Marie Sidirovsky, Editor-in-Charge, and delivered the completed manuscript with the title, *Movement Therapy for Stroke Patients*. Although this was two and a half years after the grant was received to develop the "manual," Signe's work was far from finished. Pre-publication production by Harper and Row's staff would not begin until September. A final published book would not be available for almost two more years!

On February 14, Dr. Morton Hoberman (now deceased), then Director of Rehabilitation at the New York State Rehabilitation Hospital, (now Helen Hayes Hospital,) called Signe and offered her a position as a consultant. The hospital, located in West Haverstraw, N.Y., overlooking the Hudson River, offered a complete rehabilitation service. Signe was very pleased with the potential of such a position, and after some negotiations, accepted. Part of the arrangement at the hospital was that Signe would be assigned a member of the physical therapy staff to work with her. She felt that a one-day-a-week consultancy would not be productive unless someone on the full-time staff saw to it that her Monday efforts were acted on and carried through the rest of the week. The person chosen was Kathryn A. Sawner. In a letter of January 26, 1986, Kathryn described the events:

> I was, at the time, a supervising physical therapist and was thought to be fairly well-grounded in Brunnstrom's approach to management of hemiplegia. In truth, I was probably no better grounded in her approach than most of the other staff, but was responsible for presenting her approach in the lecture series we offered the PT interns and, to that end, had done a little extra reading perhaps. One Monday morning (I remember it well!) Dr. Hoberman arrived in PT with Signe—I had no idea who she was—and asked to speak with me. From that moment, I became Signe's shadow, alter ego, organizer, and sometimes confidant. The hemiplegia text was in the middle stages of production then and I even got a bit involved with proofreading the later chapters.
>
> Getting to know Signe and working with her during our time together at Haverstraw was a wonderful experience whose memory will forever be with me, as she was the most charming, endearing, dedicated, and humble person I have ever known. That's not to say that life with Signe was always easy, for she was also demanding and somewhat irreverent about keeping to a schedule when it interfered with her first love—patients. She would demand a schedule and, in keeping with the prerogatives of those who demand, ignore it in favor of something more to her liking, invariably extending a chat with one of the staff about a particular patient, or working just an extra minute or two with a patient herself. Had I not loved and respected her thoroughly, I would undoubtedly have strangled her. Love and respect conquered all! We saw patients, gave lectures, helped others develop lectures of their own, and, during the days she wasn't with me, I struggled to

make sure her last visit was productive and that her next would be equally so.

With her commitment to Haverstraw, Signe felt it was necessary to relinquish another activity. At the end of February, she called her dear friend Ruth Dickinson at Columbia and informed her that she would be unavailable for lectures in May.

At Haverstraw, Signe also had the good fortune of working with another very competent physical therapist, Jeanne LaVigne. Jeanne was Director of Clinical Education. At one point, Signe, Kathy and Jeane decided to revise the assessment form that was included in the hemiplegia manuscript. Kathy related: "As was always true of Signe, she had no selfish interest in proclaiming that what she had once done was the best and, though inordinately stubborn at times, was always open to suggestions for improvement. Thus revising the assessment form was much to her liking if it meant a more useful product in the end." Kathy left Haverstraw to join the Department of Physical Therapy at the State University of Buffalo before the project was completed. She continued, however, to work with Signe and Jeanne, "at a distance until we were all satisfied that we had a useful, valid and reliable instrument."

Jeanne had complete access to the manuscript on hemiplegia. A student at the time at Haverstraw, Kathryn Romenski recalled seeing the material. (Today she is Director of Physical Therapy at Allied Services in Scranton, Pa.). She wrote on November 26, 1984:

> Jeanne LaVigne showed me the hand-written manuscript. I was afraid to handle such a work; ran my fingers over the cover as one would an ornate precious gold-leafed Bible. The few pages I looked through were handled like delicate rice-paper. I think I held my breath the entire experience! Couldn't wait to buy the "finished book." Made it extra special having seen and handled the original. The "rush" I experienced dealing with the manuscript made me tingle and glow with

pride in my profession and in those who made it and me/us what we are.

Throughout the spring, Signe worked on plans to build a house on the triangle of acreage still in her possession at Bullet Hole Road. At first it was a small house, and then she discovered that the building code of the town of Patterson requires "a minimum of 750 square feet for a house." Working with local builders, Signe was ready to move into her new home by July 31.

In addition to the work brought on by such a move, Signe prepared for a workshop she had agreed to present in Vermont. On October 30 she headed for Burlington, with an overnight stop in Warrensburg, N.Y. She left her motel at 6 in the morning for the Port Kent Ferry and arrived in Burlington at 11:30. She then examined and evaluated some patients at the Vermont Rehabilitation Center. In the evening she lectured with slides for two-and-a-half hours. The symposium was held November 1–3 at the University of Vermont. Signe described the success of the program:

> The workshop in Burlington was very successful and well attended by therapists of neighboring states and some 20–30 Canadian therapists and by a fellow from Thailand who expressed his hopes to see me soon—in Thailand! On my way home, I visited with a therapist, Marjory Sheldon, now retired, who lives on the family farm in Vermont now tended by her two nephews. It was a lovely farm, and I got a good night's sleep, then she showed me the farm, her riding horse, etc, and I met the two families of her nephews. She is 72 years old, but still goes horseback riding, usually accompanied by her nephew's girl on a pony. The entire drive back home through lovely farm country was most enjoyable. It is a trip which I wanted to take for many years, although I never got around to it until I had a professional engagement up there.

On November 19, Signe typed a brief letter to Major Mary Torp and included corrections to a hemiplegia classification and progress record. Referring to the hemiplegia book, Signe wrote: "The publication date is not as yet set, but I estimate that it will be a few more months before the book is ready for sale. It is a slow and tedious process." She also mentioned the move to the "triangle" house, "Finally, I have moved into my new house built on the remaining acreage, and things are looking up, although the location cannot compare with my old house. . . . "

Just before some cold weather arrived, Signe was home. She was ready to enjoy the new house. Among the features she included in the plans was a full basement under the house where the water pump, oil burner, electric water heater and the washtubs were located. It also served as a storage room, quite a luxury for Signe. In general, she was very pleased with her new home, but she soon faced many problems due to the poor-quality workmanship. The first "near-disaster" occurred after the basement floor had been cemented, and before the cement was fully dry. Due to faulty grading of the grounds, a heavy rain caused water and mud to flow through the opening in the door into the basement. According to Signe, "the water rose to about one foot in spite of the existence of a drain in the floor." When the water finally ran off, it left a great amount of mud! After waiting several days, Signe swept it a half-dozen times with and without sawdust (used to absorb the moisture). "The contractor who was responsible for the grading did nothing to help remove the mud," Signe wrote. He said, "it was unfortunate that it rained so hard."

The next problem involved a leak in the water pipes leading to the spring house. The fault was finally corrected, but it took several weeks, during which Signe kept the pump off most of the time. "After two months, I am still getting some dirt in the water, but it has gradually lessened. so that I hope finally to get clear water in the house."

Another near-disaster occurred when the hot water heater almost blew up. Signe woke up in the middle of the night from the sound of a rattling noise, and found the water tank in the basement and the pipes in the bathroom shaking vigorously as the water boiled in the tank. She described the action she took: "I ran down in the basement with a flash-light and searched for the main switch, which I fortunately found, although it had not been labelled. Much to my relief, the shaking stopped and I could eventually let out some boiling water to decrease the pressure."

In the first cold spell in October, there was another problem. When Signe started the heating system, it "made an awful noise so I turned it off again." She called the contractor, who did not have a man to send out and suggested she call the oil burner man. "This I refused to do as I found out the contractor was responsible." Signe went without heat for three days before the man from Carmel Lumber Company came to replace the faulty fuel pump. In the process, oil flowed out through the back-fill pipe which could not be controlled by a plug. Signe had to crouch on the floor to stop the oil by using her thumb as a plug, while the man removed the defective pump and installed the new one. After wiping up the mess, the repairman noticed that there still was a lot of oil on the basement floor under the chamber of the burner. He feared that an explosion would occur if she turned on the burner. Consulting by phone with the contractor, he was told, "start the burner and see what happens!" Armed with a fire extinguisher, he started the burner and no explosion occurred. Signe was not very pleased with the possibility that once the oil was heated there could be an explosion. She kept the burner off most of the time, using it sparingly to allow the oil to slowly evaporate. The smell of oil permeated the house. For safety's sake, Signe warmed the house primarily with the open fireplace and a small kerosene stove. The contractor never came around to apologize or to see how she was doing. Signe felt that after she had paid $2,000 for the job, he obviously did not care any more. How exasperating it must have been for her.

Because so much work was left unfinished in the house when the workers "rushed off," Signe worked very hard at such major chores as: "painting the outside windows before winter; cleaning out the rain water gutters; climbing up to the roof on a long ladder (before water and leaves clogged them up, this because the workers failed to come and put up the gutter screens); constructing makeshift leaders where the vertical ones had been left unfinished, etc. The work indoors, left unfinished, still remains to be done.'' She also had to collect firewood and split logs for emergency use in the fireplace, and put up a fence to protect a certain area from damage by the snowplow, ''all jobs that couldn't wait.'' All of this was described in a letter of December 18 to her sisters in Sweden. (It is important to note that, less than two weeks later Signe would be 71 years old!)

In her closing paragraph, Signe described two snowstorms that hit the area, necessitating ''snow shovelling of the driveway and entrances so as to be able to get in and out.'' Because of one storm, she had to cancel her Monday trip to the Rehabilitation Hospital. ''There is a prediction of another storm for tomorrow, so I must rush this letter to the post office before I get snow-bound again! I am therefore closing wishing all of you a restful Christmas holiday and a Happy New Year.''

Signe's former cottage, with the attached ''coop'' and the nearby barn, was still not completely demolished. She had to watch it go very slowly. How painful that must have been. Scavengers invaded the area. In her words: '' . . . the barn is a skeleton after all kinds of people have helped themselves to siding and to old oak and chestnut boards. The cottage has been robbed of its oil burner, of windows and doors, including the garage door, and all glass has been smashed for good measure. The bulldozers are expected to come to give the coup-de-grace to both buildings within a week or two. Maybe the tears will stop rolling out of my eyes when it is all over!'' It was a sad reminder of the earlier, happier days.

There was some activity on December 3 when the highway crew came and cut down some trees on Signe's side of Bullet Hole Road. ''They have also cut down trees on my former grounds including the spruce I planted in 1940 and the Blue Spruce next to the cottage.'' Trudging through the snow on December 22, Signe managed to pry loose some chestnut boards from the old barn. Perhaps it was her way of having a small memento of her good life.

Once again the holidays were spent in the company of her cousin, Nini, who came "for Christmas eve dinner and a chat." They spent New Year's Day together and welcomed 1969.

In January, Signe continued her visits to the Rehabilitation Hospital. With the encouragement of Dr. Hoberman, she met with Dr. Carpandale, the director, to discuss setting up a two-week course sometime in the spring on treatment of the hemiplegic patient. She was most pleased to have the assistance of Jeanne LaVigne and Kathy Sawner in the proposed project. The two physical therapists would work very closely with Signe from that time on.

The snow accumulation in the first week of February was "at least 24 inches, more in drifts." Jeanne and Kathy canceled a visit to Signe's house on the 9th, but were able to get through on the 12th. The meeting was held to discuss plans for two proposed workshops: one in the Rehab Hospital in Haverstraw, and another in St. Louis. In two weeks, Signe prepared a complete outline for the first workshop.

At the end of February, Signe's notes indicated, "struggle with editors at Harper & Row continues." The problems were not necessarily due to Signe's writing. David P. Miller, a former editor for the publisher, wrote on February 11, 1985:

> Since I joined Harper & Row in April 1969 and her book was published in November of 1970 it was obviously well underway by the time of my arrival. I do not recall the exact nature of the production problems that we had with the book, but they were probably in line with some of the incompetency that the Department had been experiencing at that point.

Her work on the submitted manuscript was far from finished.

Signe was always known to be a strong and dynamic individual. Whatever weaknesses she may have had were rarely, if ever, seen in public. She was an individual who kept things, especially problems, to herself. The loss of her home and grounds at Bullet Hole was probably the most distressing occurrence in her life. The devastating blow took place on

March 10. Signe wrote in her notes: " . . . came home from West Haverstraw. Cottage had been erased by a bulldozer, was set on fire, no watchman in view. Fire had spread to the barn and sparks were flying toward spring house. Fires burned all night. At 9 P.M. watchman came, said he would stop burning of the barn."

Once again, in correspondence (April 28, 1969) to her sisters, Signe described her "trials and tribulations at the Bullet Hole:"

> During February and March, I saw the demolishment and burning of my former home, the two-hundred year old barn, and the old farmhouse. There is now not a sign of anything, except that the tree stump of the wonderful Linden tree was pushed up toward my property the other day, and it still hurts to see it. Blasting, intensive, has been going on since the middle of March. Massive heaps of crushed rocks have been dumped on my beautiful lawn. Trucks as big as house and evil-looking bulldozers make deafening noise from early in the morning to late at night. Three to four times a week when a big blast goes off, a man comes to tell me that I have to get out of the house, because "it is cheaper to repair houses than to kill people." So I take the dogs in the car and drive away a considerable distance, where I have to sit and wait, sometimes a whole hour, before I hear the blast. What a nuisance, and the days I am away from home I am terribly worried about the dogs. They get so frightened that they even refuse to eat. So far, my new house has not been hit by rocks, but one of the other houses in this area was struck twice, a big rock went through the roof, cracked one of the main beams and landed in the living room. I have taken down my mirrors from the walls and been told to stay away from the windows. How long will this all go on? "Well, we will be around all Summer" was the answer.

Perhaps the final clearance of the land had some benefit, as Signe indicated she felt better "now that my old home has disappeared from the map." She took up more interest in her new house and once again worked around the yard and garden. As to hiring any help, Signe was able to find one man for a half-day. He was Mr. Simpson, age 75. "I don't dare to ask him to do the heavy work," she wrote, "as he is rather stubborn, so his usefulness for me is minimal." That left the heavy work to 71-year-old Signe!

As of March 28, no payment had been made by the state for the land and building appropriated two years before. Signe consulted Mr. Costello, a lawyer, to see how the payment could be expedited. Evidently, the final payment depended upon Signe obtaining an "easement" from a neighbor who was not readily available. On April 28, Signe obtained the release which opened the way for the State to process her check. The check from the Division of Taxation and Finance, Department of the Treasury, dated June 11, 1969, arrived on July 3. It was for $11,542.50. There was an overpayment of $135, which Signe noted would be deducted from the final settlement. The corrected amount that Signe accepted was $11,407.50. She received an additional amount of $5,641.75 on September 8.

Four days later, Signe was off for Seattle to participate in the two-week workshop on hemiplegia. Almost immediately upon arrival on the 13th, Signe met with the workshop faculty at the North West Hospital. Included in the group were Ann McWilliam, Fritz Johnson, Martha Trotter, Darlene Herteling, Wilma Footh, and Frederic Harris.

Before starting the workshop, Signe wanted to see one of the most famous natural sites in the area. She met some old friends, Gudrun and Carolyn Tauberg, and they took her to see Mt. Rainier.

Jeanne LaVigne, Kathy Sawner and a senior student from the University of Buffalo, Stuart MacRoberts, arrived on Sunday in order to serve as faculty for the workshop. They weren't surprised at all to learn that 71-year-old Signe was out climbing Mt. Rainier. Kathy recalled that Signe "was the absolute personification of vigor. We did a two-week workshop on that trip plus a Saturday program in between. Stu, Jeanne, and I were exhausted on Sunday, our only free day, but Signe once again donned her walking shoes to pursue the mountain. We held her in awe.''

Stuart's participation in the program was unique. He had jokingly said to Kathy that ''perhaps she needed a helper'' at the workshop, and with Signe's permission arrangements were made. Before leaving for Seattle, Stuart and Kathy spent a great amount of time practicing on patients at the Buffalo VA Hospital.

Kathy, Jeanne and Stuart met with Signe in Seattle before the workshop to work out assignments. Stuart recalled in a letter of January 13, 1986, that he was to ''act as a helper during the lectures and to participate as a group leader during the lab sessions.'' Even though he still was a PT student, in Seattle he led a group of experienced therapists and all went well.

Stuart also accompanied Signe on evaluation rounds, looking for patients to use in the labs. On one occasion, Signe evaluated a patient and found very little or no elbow extensor in the prone position. ''I asked Signe if I could try,'' Stuart related, ''and managed to get a much better response from the patient. Stuart remembers how Signe complimented him and ''made me feel so good about that and gave me the feeling of actually being of use.'' He also marveled at how well Signe could motivate patients to try. ''She had a wonderful ability to get the very most out of patients and leave them feeling good about themselves. She never tried to push a patient beyond his/her capability and certainly never asked for an action that the patient did not have some chance of achieving.''

The workshop was held September 15–26. One of the local physical therapists who was involved with the program was Bud Haley. Now in Modesto, California, with the Gold Bear Physical Therapy Services, Bud recalled his meeting with Signe in a letter of July 28, 1984:

> At the time she was presenting her course on stroke rehabilitation, she asked the local therapists to provide

> some difficult patients so that she could demonstrate her techniques. I was awed by her presence and at the same time somewhat skeptical when I saw the patients she had to deal with. In short, I was amazed at what happened. In just a few minutes she had the patients doing things the therapists had not been able to accomplish in weeks of trying. I asked myself how could this be? Was she more skilled? Was she psychic? Or was it something else? My conclusion then and something I still believe today was that she had a unique manner with people; a personality trait that said ''you can do it.'' There was a twinkle in her eye and tone in her voice that made the patient perk up. To this day I have tried to emulate these qualities in my work. I feel that a large part of my success is a direct result of my brief encounter with Miss Brunnstrom.

On Friday evening, Kathy, Jeanne, Stuart and some of the local therapists went to the ''best'' oriental restaurant for dinner. It took more than an hour to be seated and more than that for the meal. The next morning, the ''faculty'' was to participate in an all-day workshop with unlimited registration. On the way back to the motel, the group was worried that Signe would be mad because of the late hour. She wanted to review with Kathy and Jeanne how the program would be handled. It was 10:30 when they arrived at Signe's room. Stuart recalled that there Signe was, sitting on her bed, hemming up a dress. ''The one that she was going to wear was not new,'' he recalled, and was of an old style coming below her knees. Signe went into the bathroom, put on the dress, and came out and asked for my approval! She was more worried about how she would look than anything else.

Another humorous situation developed at breakfast. Jeanne made some comment that led to her saying, ''Miss Brunnstrom, with a mind like that, you really could go far.'' Signe thoroughly enjoyed that and thought it was very funny. Afterwards, Stuart often would use that comment just to make her laugh.

During the workshop, Stuart's responsibility included handling the "2 x 2" lantern slides. A large projector was used, and he had to change the slides. Suddenly, bubbles started to develop in the slide because of the heat. "I felt terrible," he remarked, "pulling slides out as Signe was trying to illustrate a point . . . but it kept her moving in the lectures. A year or so later, Stuart had some of the slides copied in 35mm format, but he did not finish the job before he left the area. Signe had someone else complete the project, and being the person she was, she sent a complete set to Stuart for his own use.

With the workshop over, Kathy and Stuart went back to Buffalo. Stuart knew he had gone to Seattle with no expectation of payment, but a few weeks later Kathy called him into her office, and he was presented with a check for $200 as a gift from an anonymous donor. Years later, Kathy admitted that the money was a gift from Miss Brunnstrom "to help him out. . .but she didn't want him to know."

After graduation, Stuart and his wife Kris visited Signe at Bullet Hole Road on several occasions. They would always call first to see if she was busy. Signe, while she enjoyed their visit, always reminded them to eat before they came, "as she was not planning lunch."

After Seattle, arriving home on September 27, Signe went back to work on her various projects, while suffering the inconveniences of the continuous blasting from the road construction. Her work included: three days "working on the ditch for rain water"; meeting with Jeanne LaVigne to review the program for another workshop at the State Rehab Hospital; building a stone wall by the well house; attending a meeting of the Professional Advisory Committee of the Putnam County Department of Health's Home Health Agency; reading Mary Taylor's research report; shoveling some six inches of snow; and reviewing a new format for the pages of the hemiplegia book, requested by Harper and Row. Signe was indefatigable!

She also was always ready to work with students. G. Gordon Williamson was an occupational therapy student at Columbia. He now is Director of the Pediatric Rehabilitation Department at John F. Kennedy Medical Center's Johnson Institute in Edison, New Jersey. On May 5, 1985, he wrote:

> I first met Signe in 1969 when two carloads of occupational therapy students, Simmie Cynkin (our instructor) and Ruth Dickinson (then Assistant Director of the Physical Therapy program) visited her in Putnam County at her home. She was a very gracious hostess showing us her house and grounds in a lovely wooded setting. Signe was an athletic individual who thoroughly enjoyed the outdoors. I was struck at the time by her honest, direct manner that had no trace of pretense or affectation. For such an accomplished individual that is a rare and wonderful quality.
>
> Before that time I knew of Signe through her writing. I had read her textbook in my Kinesiology class and was currently studying her therapeutic approach to hemiplegia using a pre-publication manual. The manual was so beautifully written that I was teaching myself the approach during my fieldwork placement at the Rusk Institute of Rehabilitation Medicine, New York University Medical Center.
>
> The afternoon with Signe was spent discussing the evaluation and treatment of hemiplegia. She talked with great enthusiasm and freshness on the topic. It impressed me that one could be near the end of a long and productive career and still be intellectually and personally excited about clinical issues. In her modesty she challenged us to view her contribution as only a beginning and to develop our thinking further. An inquisitive mind is never content with current answers.

Before Thanksgiving, from November 12 through 24, Signe was a major participant in the workshop presented at the New York State Rehabilitation Hospital. Working with Kathy Sawncr and Jeanne LaVigne, the program demonstrated that Signe still had the energy and stamina to do a full day's work of teaching over the two-week period.

In Signe's diary, for December 2, there is an interesting notation, "Japanese translation of 'Clinical Kinesiology' arrived from F.A. Davis, Co."

As Christmas approached, Signe still could be found working on revisions of the hemiplegia book. Once again, her cousin Nini came to spend New Year's Day, 1970, with her. Another birthday!

In the first two weeks of January, 1970, Signe's attention was centered on the hemiplegia book. It soon became obvious that work on the book would take a lot of her time. She prepared a list for Harper & Row of people who were to be sent promotional material. Galley proofs arrived on January 9, and by the 15th they were corrected. Several days later, Signe worked on abstracts of the galleys and made comments for the editor. Before the end of January, Signe had the layout or "cut-dummy" of chapters one to five. In the first week of February, she completed her examination of the illustrations and legends through Chapter Six. In spite of the inclement winter weather, Signe went to the city and met with Miss Kovner and the designer of the book in the publisher's office on 23rd Street. Signe's work was far from finished.

On May 21, it was decided that a new promotional piece had to be prepared. She still had more page proofs to review and the index had to be completed. Carrying her entire set of index cards, she made another trip to the city on July 20 for a conference with the editors. Her notes indicate that as late in the year as July 31, she was working on the index. In the first two weeks of August, Signe "struggled with the index and unreasonable editors and promoters." By September 18, page proofs of the index arrived. Finally, in mid-November, the good news came from Harper & Row that the book was in publication! It would be three months before Signe would see the final result of her five years of work.

In between the work on the book, Signe assisted a physical therapist, Ellen Blodgett of Ft. Montgomery, who worked for the Putnam County Department of Health. On February 27, Signe wrote, "Started to accompany Ellen Blodgett for home treatment of stroke patients." Ms.

Blodgett recalled (April 2, 1985) Signe assisted her with treating a CVA patient in Brewster. She also visited Signe at Bullet Hole and learned how independent she was in managing her home and grounds. "I attempted to help her as much as she needed but Signe was a 'jack-of-all trades' person!"

Signe seemed so preoccupied with her new home that she cut down on her travel. The Canadian Physical Therapy Association held its conference March 12–13 in Toronto, but Signe felt she was unable to participate, and asked Kathy Sawner to represent her.

The major professional responsibility Signe maintained involved weekly trips to the State Rehab Hospital to meet with instructors and outline "practice sessions" in preparation for a workshop planned in early May.

On March 17, Signe heard that Mrs. Lang, her former neighbor and the original owner of the Bullet Hole property, was in the hospital. The very next day, Signe was at her bedside for a visit. She visited her several times, until April 14 when Mrs. Lang was transferred to the Tree Haven Nursing Home. At this point, Signe's notes indicate how generous she had been for a long period of time, "Social Service takes over, no longer any need to give Mrs. Lang $60 per month as I had done for many years." Signe never discussed her financial contributions to her friend, but just assumed the responsibility in her own kind and inimitable way.

Throughout the next five months, Signe was quite concerned over the illness of her cousin, Nini. Despite having her own problems, Signe devoted much time to doing many things for her cousin. During this period, work on the hemiplegia book continued.

With the book almost completed, another project developed. On July 29, Signe received a call from Joe Witcher of F.A. Davis Company, asking for a revision of *Clinical Kinesiology*. Signe was amenable to the revision, but the publisher wanted it to be completed by December. She was not about to undertake such a task and came up with two brilliant possible solutions. One would be to havc a very competent clinical educator who was teaching kinesiology serve as the editor of the third revision. Signe wrote that she had been "concentrating on neurophysiological aspects of human motion with reference to movement therapy in hemiplegia and was no longer up to date on recent anatomical and biomechanical material." She also indicated that, "after I discontinued teaching the Kinesiology course at P & S (Physicians and Surgeons, Columbia University), I lost contact with students and could no longer take advantage of their comments and attitudes with regards to the course contents." Signe felt Ruth Dickinson of Columbia would be the ideal person to revise the material.

The other idea was to "donate" the assignment of the book to the APTA, with the accompanying responsibility of any revisions in accordance with the original contract. On the very day that Mr. Witcher called, Signe typed a letter to Mary Elizabeth Kolb, the Associate Executive Director of APTA:

> One of the matters I had planned to discuss with you before you moved to Washington, D.C. was in regard to my book *Clinical Kinesiology* which was first published in 1962 and which has sold increasingly well since then. The 2nd edition appeared in 1966 and in 1968 there was a reprint of 5,000 copies which supply will soon be exhausted.
>
> I would like to assign the contract for the book to the APTA which would mean that the APTA gets the benefit of the royalties which lately have amounted to well over $1,000 a year. However, some responsibilities go with such assignment, as specified in the enclosed original contract. Please refer this matter to whatever committee handles such affairs.

Signe suggested that, "if the assignment would go into effect soon, the APTA would have to provide funds for the revision." She also felt that someone familiar with the book, specifically a kinesiology instructor, would be best-suited to do the revision. If the APTA did not accept her offer, whoever was to do the revision would have her name on the new text and share in the royalties with Signe.

Royce Noland, the APTA Executive Director, wrote Signe on August 5, raising some questions about the responsibility of the new assignee and how the most competent person would be found to do the revision. Signe responded in a letter of August 15, emphasizing that "the responsibilities following assignment are quite clearly outlined in the contract." She then suggested that in order to relieve APTA of the responsibility of finding the competent individual to revise the book, "and because time is running short," she had communicated with a colleague in New York City asking her to revise the book. "I sincerely hope that she will respond in the affirmative," Signe said referring to Ruth Dickinson.

On September 1, Ruth called Signe and indicated she would be interested in preparing the third edition, but it could not be ready by December 30. Two weeks later, Signe received the following letter from Royce Noland:

> I have discussed your kind proposal on the assignment of the contract in reference to your book with President Michels. He has done some investigation on the posture of the Board of Directors in reference to such activity and has found that it would be, assuming the contract with its responsibilities, inconsistent with the policies of the Board.
>
> We certainly appreciate your offer, but Mr. Michels and I both agree that it is not feasible for us to accept.

Much to Signe's delight, on September 16, Ruth was at the new house on Bulletin Hole Road to discuss the revision. Even though Signe would assist in the revision, Ruth indicated it could not be completed by the F.A. Davis deadline of December 30. Within a few days, Signe was at the State Rehabilitation Hospital library collecting references for the third edition. "I have collected articles on locomotion which I want to read," she wrote Ruth on September 28. "I also found some kinesiology articles which you may want to glance through for possible use in Clinical Kinesiology." She also gave Ruth some advice: " . . . would suggest that you now determine the style of the bibliography you wish to use in the 3rd ed. in terms of capitalization, use of initials of authors, etc. and that you confer with Mr. Witcher about the style preferred by the publisher. It will save you much work later, if you write correct bibliography cards as you go along.'' While Signe was most willing to have Ruth do the third edition, it was obvious that she was not quite ready to give up her complete involvement in seeing it come to fruition.

Bonnie Blossom, now in Atlanta, was Director of Physical Therapy at the hospital from August, 1970, through 1974. She recalled in a letter of November 20, 1984, how she often saw Signe:

> I caught a whisper of her here and a glimpse of her there when she visited the hospital. When she came to use the library or other resources, she did so as though she was entering a church. She did not want to inconvenience or be in the way. She was so shy about her contributions to physical therapy. She clearly was caught up in her thought process and had little to no interest in the recognition and honor that went with it. She was out to solve problems and to share her resolutions with others . . . that was her mission.

Signe also was not to be forgotten as a teacher. Physical and occupational therapists still wanted to participate in continuing education programs in which she demonstrated treatment techniques applied to the hemiplegic patient. Cecila Satterly, O.T., wrote Signe on September 21, inviting her to participate in an occupational therapy institute scheduled for April 12, 1971, at the State University of New York at Downstate, Brooklyn. Planning for the workshop involved several meetings and a trip to the Downstate Center on October 15. Two days later, the planning committee met at Signe's home.

In late October, Signe prepared for a visit from her sisters. When Elsa and Ingegerd arrived, they were treated to the local sights in Signe's Ford Falcon. She drove them to Bear Mountain, West Point, Pond Ridge, and together they all visited Mrs. Lang in the nursing home. A workshop was scheduled at the Rehabilitation Hospital in West Haverstraw, but Signe stayed with her family and left "Kathy and Jeanne in charge."

Signe was also invited to attend some clinical conferences at the Harlem Hospital Center. She felt she could not go and asked Althea Jones if she could cover the sessions. Althea agreed to the assignment.

For Signe's 73rd birthday, 1970 ended with "heavy snow at night!"

The weather kept Signe at home, but not idle. In between shoveling snow, she worked on abstracts for inclusion in the third revision of *Clinical Kinesiology*.

Ten copies of *Movement Therapy in Hemiplegia* arrived "finally" on February 9, 1971, from Harper & Row. At long last, Signe was able to enjoy the fruits of her labor. She decided that personally-autographed copies would be sent to certain select people. Among those were Ginnete Elmiger in Germany, Andre Albert of France, Dr. Herbert Elftman, Anthony DeRosa and Jack Hofkosh.

Working with Ruth on the revisions project in early February, Signe wrote Mr. Witcher at F.A. Davis regarding the style-guide to be used in the third edition. She also corresponded with Pat Murray, Chief of the Kinesiological Research Laboratory at the VA Center in Milwaukee. Signe wrote Pat on February 12, asking for some reprints on a gait study of normal women. Pat responded on February 18, indicating, "We will be honored to have you mention our studies in your excellent kinesiology text." Pat thought it would be interesting to see how Signe would use her material, but demonstrating her trust in Signe, she wrote, "I have often commented on your scholarly approach in reporting scientific literature and therefore feel no need to check whatever you may say about our studies."

Another meeting was held on February 24 at Columbia to plan the OT workshop. Those present included Althea Jones, Sigrid Hansen, Kathy Sawner and G. Gordon Williamson. Signe and Kathy also discussed invitations to conduct workshops in Memphis and in Puerto Rico.

Throughout March, Signe continued planning the OT institute set for April 12. Signe typed 50 reference cards to be used in the course. During the institute, Signe noted, "a male patient asked, where is the chief mechanic . . . the one who knows how we are put together?"

G. Gordon Williamson described his role in the institute:

> I had the good fortune of serving as a lab assistant to Signe. It was a great honor to be chosen as one of her instructors, and I was thrilled and hesitant at the same time. After all I had only one year's experience behind me. But Signe was supportive, and quickly I felt at ease. The highlight of the conference was watching her work with patients. Now that was a treat. As one would expect she had impeccable skills in analyzing movements, grading treatment, and therapeutic handling. She and Berta Bobath will go down in history in that category. However, what really made an impression was Signe's ability to understand and relate to the patients as individuals. Her communication with them was palpable. She had a way of personalizing her therapy so that they were motivated and felt competent. The old adage of working from strengths and not weakness was put into practice. This tremendous gift is rather surprising in that Signe had a distinct Scandinavian accent which could have been a barrier. Instead it gave her character that matched her quick and warm smile.

Stu MacRoberts also was involved with the Downstate workshop. He was used as a model during the demonstration and recalled an amusing incident. Signe had Stu in front of the audience to illustrate the proper way to facilitate the Searratus Anterior. Stu wrote: "I have fairly obvious winging Scapula. As Signe began the demonstration, she realized that anatomical fact and pointed it out to everyone." Her Swedish accent came into play when she said, "you have VINGING scapula," and everyone thought that was quite funny at the time!

On April 29, Ruth Dickinson visited with Signe to confer about the revision. Signe noted Ruth "made good progress, but much remains to be done." In another letter to Ruth, on May 4, Signe pointed out the need for some additional references related to "the soleus as a knee flexor in late stance phase. I am in the process of re-reading the entire Locomotion Chapter and will let you know if I find anything else of importance to be corrected." She ended the brief letter to Ruth with the comment: "I enjoyed your visit with me. It is always nice talking to you."

At last Signe received some financial remuneration for all the time spent on the hemiplegic book. A check for $321.46 arrived on April 28 from Harper & Row, representing the "balance of royalties ending December 30, 1970."

On the weekend of May 10, 1971, Highway 84 was opened for traffic. This was an event Signe did not look forward to. She heard trucks "day and night." It was the culmination of the highway construction that destroyed the peace and tranquility Signe so desperately longed for!

In May, Signe received an invitation to give the Mary McMillan lecture at the next APTA meeting in Cleveland. As she had done previously, she again refused the honor. There is no explanation in her notes for the action.

Another letter, May 25, indicated the manuscript was completed, as Signe congratulated Ruth on the third edition. "Few people realize," she wrote, "what a tremendous job was involved, but I do." She also suggested the publisher could engage someone to do the indexing after the page proofs were ready."

Recognizing the important work Ruth Dickinson did with the third edition of *Clinical Kinesiology*, Signe offered to assign the contract with F.A. Davis directly to Ruth. She wanted Ruth to personally have the contract, and not the university, for fear that the donation "would be swallowed up by the administration." Signe told Ruth she wanted the assignment to be made before the new edition was actually distributed so that "the royalty for that edition goes to you." That gesture was a true demonstration of the friendship Signe had for Ruth Dickinson.

Signe next faced a major problem with her dog, Kaya. Over several weeks, Kaya had seizures for short durations. Medicine was prescribed, but did not help. By mid-June, Kaya's hind limbs were weak. Signe sat for hours on the lawn with Kaya, often until the sun went down. On July 15 at 5:30, Signe noticed that Kaya's condition had worsened. She described what happened:

> Kaya stayed in her basket. She followed me with her eyes wherever I went. I will never forget her expression. Nini came, we took Kaya to Dr. Thomas, carried her in her basket to the car. She stayed quiet, but her eyes were wide open. Nini waited in the doctor's waiting room until it was all over. She said she heard Kaya stretch. Back home, I took Rebel for a walk feeling miserable. For a year or more I felt as if I had betrayed Kaya and constantly felt her eyes following me. Could not sleep and had difficulties concentrating, even at workshops in Memphis, cried every night there.

The Memphis workshop, arranged by Ray Patterson, started on August 15. Signe arrived at 5 the day before and stayed at the Sheraton Motor Inn (the room cost $10 a day). In the first week, the course was for student physical therapists, and in the second week, only practicing therapists were admitted. Once again, Signe had the formidable assistance of Kathy Sawner and Jeanne LaVigne. While in Memphis, Signe took the sightseeing trip on the "Queen of Memphis" along the Mississippi. The workshop program ended with a banquet at the Faculty Club. Arriving at La Guardia Airport, Signe took a cab to Grand Central Station and the train to Brewster.

In September, Signe made a decision to sell the new "triangle" house. The highway noise was too much for her. Throughout the month, she used her new, white, two-door Ford Maverick (purchased at a cost of $2,422, including extras and sales tax,) to search for a new apartment or house. She found one in the basement of someone's home with a rent of $180 per month—"too much, apartment dark." She decided to keep looking and to try a rental agent.

October 5 was a good day! A royalty check arrived from Harper & Row for $2,415.15, "much more than I expected," according to Signe's notes. Added to earlier payments of $4,291.49 from H & R and $1,175.85 from F.A. Davis, the total royalties "came to $5,467 for both books." This included payments for books sold prior to January 1, 1972.

Signe was now determined to see that the assignment papers giving *Clinical Kinesiology* to Ruth were completed. On October 7, a letter was sent to Robert Craven, President of F.A. Davis (with a copy to Ruth,) in which Signe detailed how the assignment would be passed to Ruth. She wrote:

> Miss Dickinson is a very capable person who has taught kinesiology for a considerable number of years and who keeps abreast with new developments in the field. She presently is preparing the 3rd edition of the book which is almost ready to go to press. I am very happy that Miss Dickinson has agreed to take over the responsibilities for the book. She is of course entitled to the royalties for the 3rd edition and also for future editions, if any. I would suggest that she receive the royalties for all sales after January 1, 1972.

Although six months had passed since the death of her dog, Signe still missed her friend very much. On December 2, Signe sent a contribution of $50 to the Putnam County Humane Society "in memory of my beloved dog, Kaya, who lived until she was 18, her last day was July 15. She was the best friend I ever had."

In the closing weeks of 1971, Signe completed the transactions that would give the assignment rights of her two very popular books to her dear friends, Kathy Sawner and Ruth Dickinson. The assignments would include the transfer of all future royalties. Kathy would have *Movement Therapy in Hemiplegia* and Ruth received *Clinical Kinesiology*. The final contract and assignment "of the 3rd edition (Clinical Kinesiology) and all subsequent editions" was signed on December 30, 1971, by Robert Craven, John Paul Dalsimer, Ruth Dickinson and Signe Brunnstrom.

Kathy recalled:

> Signe hated loose ends, as those who knew her were well aware, and saw me as a person in whom she could entrust her 'state-side' hemiplegia efforts. I have believed for some time that she was trying to prepare me for this from our very first day together. I don't recall the first time she mentioned passing along the hemiplegia text to me, but I well recall shying away from it for a long time before I finally acceded to her wishes. She was so grateful and I realized only then that I had caused her much agony by my persistent refusals. This 'gesture' paved the way for her return to Sweden in 1973.

In a letter of December 9, Harper and Row Publisher David P. Miller, stated, "May I please urge you to discuss this matter with your own lawyer or tax consultant, due to the nature and magnitude of this agreement and the effect it will have upon your own personal affairs." Signe had made her decision. The assignment to Kathy was signed on December 23 and became effective on January 1, 1972. Signe would receive no further royalties from her two popular texts.

The year 1971 ended with a holiday visit to Mrs. Lang in the nursing home and the notation in Signe's diary, "I saw a deer, a beautiful young doe walking up our private road then running across Mrs. Olson's property."

Chapter Eight

The Twilight Years

Signe continued to look for new living quarters in January, 1972. She saw a five-room cottage priced at $25,000, but was shocked at the "mini-rooms." Accompanied by her niece, Elsa Diehl, they also saw a three-room house for rent on Peaceable Hill Road. "The place was messy," Signe wrote, "but will be cleaned up." The house would be available March 1. She decided to give the owner, Mrs. DiDio, a $20 binder.

To sell her "triangle" home on Bullet Hole Road, Signe placed an ad in the Patent Trader offering the house for $24,000. During the next to weeks, people came to see the house "more or less interested in buying, but the highway noise discouraged them." Numerous real estate people called and offered to list the house, but Signe said, "I do not approve."

On March 14, Signe made a decision and paid an additional $200 to Mrs. DiDio as security for rental of the "Peaceable Hill" house.

Fortunately, just about the same time, Mr. Harry Bates of Mahopac came to see the "triangle" house and was very interested in purchasing it. In a letter of January 20, 1986, Bates recalled the days in 1972 when he sought to purchase Signe's little house:

> Others were interested and even though I could not offer as much as some, she decided her house was just right for me and my son and while realizing a substantial money loss, chose me as the purchaser, a gesture unheard of even then. I can distinctly remember one day when we came to see her, she showed us all the land that the State had taken and then commented, "this rocky corner is all they left for me." Surely the loss of her home and land must have been a traumatic experience. Miss Brunnstrom was a trusting person. I had asked her permission to bring my parents on the weekend to see the house. She agreed, but when we got there Miss Brunnstrom was not there. She had not forgotten our visit, however. All the doors were left unlocked so we could enter freely. Is this not a "special lady?" In the short time of our acquaintance I found her to be a gentle, kind and understanding lady.

By April 5, Bates gave Signe $2,300 toward the sale price. Signe deposited the money, together with an additional $523 in royalties from F.A. Davis Company, in a new account at the Putnam County Savings Bank. She also went to her accountant to pick up her completed tax forms. (For 1971, Signe paid $946 in federal taxes and $218 in state taxes.) She also paid the first installment for the 1972 estimated tax of $237. "I objected to Mr. Romberg about the high estimated tax," she wrote, "because I knew my income for 1972 would be much smaller, owing to assignments of royalties for the books to Ruth D. and Kathy S. as of January 1, 1972, but Romberg refused to change the estimated tax."

With a closure date of April 20 set for Mr. Bates to take over her house, Signe spent her time "cleaning my house and moving furniture to Peaceable Hill Rd., sanding floors in the rented house etc." Her notes indicated she also gave many things away:

> Left some furniture to new owner and lent him a folding bed; to Leary family, antique old American chest of drawers, painting, buttersack; Navy chest for

Sarah; old school bench for boy; small ladder, roller, garden tools etc. Bench from porch stored with Leary's. To Ackermans, slates (flagstones). To Blatz, 2 wedges, one sledge hammer.

Ruth Dickinson and Charlotte Ritter visited Signe on April 16 at "an almost empty house." Together they drove to see the new place, but only from the outside. The next day, Signe completed the move. For the closing on the "triangle house," on April 20, Signe met her attorney, Mr.Costello, and Mr. Bates at the Mahopac branch of the Putnam County Federal Savings and Loan Association. She turned the house keys over to Bates and that ended 32 years of association with Bullet Hole Road.

Signe was now 74 years old. She had wonderful memories of the Bullet Hole Road area with the barn, the coop, the gardens, the cottage and her last home. She saw the landscape change from an isolated area to several homes and a major highway intersecting the land. It must have been very depressing, but with Signe's strength of character, she was determined to continue her life and try to participate in some professional activities. Kathy Sawner felt Signe "mourned her loss and never really got over it." Kathy believed all the problems connected with the loss of her home triggered Signe's thoughts "about returning to Sweden to live out the rest of her life."

On May 2, Signe received a telephone call from William Reed of the State Department in Washington in reference to a conference on neurological rehabilitation set for Rio de Janeiro in November. He wanted to know if she received a letter of invitation. Possibly because of the recent move, she did not have the letter. Reed explained the invitation would be from Professor Araujo Leitao, President of the Brazilian Congress of Neurological Rehabilitation, and include an offer to cover all expenses in Rio. Signe was to give four to eight lectures and demonstrations on motor rehabilitation of hemiplegic patients. While she was honored to be invited, Signe decided against undertaking such a venture, and when the invitation did arrive, the information was forwarded to

Kathy Sawner. Kathy made arrangements to participate in the conference in November, 1972. Her travel plans were well under way when Professor Leitao wrote indicating that "due to poor management of the Congress, the meeting had to be postponed." Kathy never heard from him again.

On May 21, Signe received a letter from Susan Freed of the Woodrow Wilson Rehabilitation Center in Fishersville, Virginia, inviting her to conduct a hemiplegia workshop. Signe gave it considerable thought, but eventually decided not to participate. The information was passed on to Kathy Sawner and the workshop was held. Kathy recalled that program as possibly being the first time she had complete responsibility for a program, "I don't remember if that was the first time she put 'Kathy in charge', but it might well have been."

The third edition, revised printing of *Clinical Kinesiology*, (revision by Ruth Dickinson,) arrived on May 12. That was just 22 months from the July 29, 1970 call from the publisher asking for the revision. In the Preface to the text, Ruth wrote:

> In this third edition, those sections of the book which represent the major contributions Miss Brunnstrom has given to our understanding of normal and abnormal kinesiology are unchanged. One of the pertinent changes made in this edition is the revision of the section in Chapter One concerned with basic mechanical principles.

She also referred to recent anatomical, electromyographic and clinical studies that had been added to the book. The Preface concludes with the statement that, "the organization of the book, which served so well in the previous editions, remains essentially the same." The price of the third edition was $7.50. Sales must have been very good, as there were second and third printings in 1973!

Ruth, accompanied by Althea Jones, visited Signe on July 5. As a demonstration of her affection, Signe gave Ruth a maple salad bowl from Vermont and several publications. These included a 1928 first edition of Wilhelmina Wright's

Muscle Function; an original copy of the University of California locomotion studies completed after World War II; the two-volume set in German of Rudolph Fick's *Anatomie und Mechanick der Gelenke*; and a variety of anatomy atlases (mostly in German). Althea was given a green, handmade Canadian vase, and a Mexican ceramic plate and 56 "two-by-two" slides prepared by the Crew Studios for Signe's lectures.

During July and August, Signe just enjoyed what garden she had and occupied her time with many errands. She drove to the Rehab Hospital "with a load of books and journals for the library"; talked to Bonnie Blossom and Tricia Sullivan; had a visit from cousin Nini; spoke to Harvey Margolin, a physical therapist in Carmel, and arranged to see him; and completed an application and had photos taken for a new passport.

Rebel, Signe's dog, also received a lot of attention, as she was getting old and the heat bothered her. Signe described the care she gave the sick animal, "wet compresses to cool her. Repeated at midnight—good results."

After the summer months, there was a sudden spurt of professional activities again. Signe received a phone call from Dr. Harriet Gillette on September 7, in reference to a possible workshop in Chicago for April, 1973. Jeanne LaVigne came for a visit on September 23 to discuss and receive "advice about an article on hemiplegia assessment." In October and November, Signe received mail: from Carol Ann Parr of the Child Development Institute at Chapel Hill, North Carolina; from a group in Puerto Rico about a workshop; and from the OT Association in Pennsylvania. The mailman brought Signe a check for $534 on October 6 as a royalty payment. She returned the check informing F.A. Davis Company that all royalties were now to be forwarded to Ruth Dickinson. Also on the sixth, her cousin visited once more, just before she started a drive south for the winter. It would be the last time Signe would see her.

Throughout December, Signe organized her papers. She sent her neurophysiology files to Kathy and Althea. The only visitor she had around Christmas was her niece. Signe continued to complain about the vehicle noises and expressed her unhappiness with the rented house. In her mind, she was getting ready to return to Sweden.

The year ended on a sad note. Cousin Nini passed away December 25 at Birmingham Hospital in Alabama. New Year's Eve was quiet for Signe, alone with just memories of the days spent with her cousin. It must have been a depressing time for this gallant lady to usher in 1973 and note her 75th birthday.

Much of the information in this publication has been based on the actual diary-like index cards maintained by Signe. However, no record of her daily or weekly activities is available for the period after 1973. Her story continues, based on letters, documents and personal comments made by those who knew her.

According to Kathryn Sawner, Signe spoke to her about a "short trip" to Sweden in January, 1973. She made the trip on March 15. She and Kathy were in San Juan at the time, and she left there for Kennedy Airport to board her flight to Stockholm. In Stockholm, she visited with her sister, Ingegered, and in Lund with her older sister, Elsa.

It was while in Lund that Signe met Kerstin Lundbladh, a Senior lecturer in the Department of Physical Therapy at the University of Lund. Kerstin recalled the incident vividly in a letter of June 3, 1986:

> I was working at the Rehabilitation unit at the University Hospital of Lund. One evening I stayed on late for some reason and as I was leaving I was approached by two elderly ladies. One of them said she was looking for a physiotherapist to whom she could introduce her sister from the United States, Signe Brunnstrom.
>
> Swedish physical therapists at the time knew of Signe Brunnstrom though her books, principally *Clinical Kinesiology*. I was aware that she had trained in Sweden and had spent virtually all her working life in the United States, but otherwise I knew nothing about her.

I was rather taken aback at our first encounter, when she abruptly came to the point. 'Are there any hemiplegic patients here? I intend moving to Sweden, I will settle in either Lund, where my eldest sister lives or in Stockholm where I have another sister. The deciding factor is my access to hemiplegic patients, not my preference of sisters.'

At the moment I could assure her of the general availability of such patients, since I would clearly need to discuss her proposals with administrative and professional colleagues before allowing her access to patients. I did ask her to demonstrate her method to the physical therapists at the hospital the following day. She was delighted to do so providing she could speak English. Coincidentally, we had an English patient in the rehab unit and I shall always remember the extraordinary contact that Signe was able to establish. She also delivered a lecture to the physiotherapy students before returning to the United States the next day. I could not be certain whether she would really return to her homeland after an absence of fifty years, and no arrangement was made between us prior to her departure.

Signe was so individual, not least in the way she spoke Swedish. I was impressed by the lack of an accent, and I was fascinated by her use of the style last heard in the 1930s. I was unsure at the time whether she was aware of it, but she later became very annoyed when she discovered her written Swedish was no longer in use.

Upon her return to the states, Signe told Kathy about her experience at the university and mentioned, "how good it was to see her sisters after so many years."

It was now late spring of 1973. Signe was very much aware that her active professional life had to be curtailed. She was ill with "stomach pains," and did not enjoy the thought of traveling extensively. It was time for retirement. She could not manage by herself. On April 25, she left

Peaceable Hill and moved to her niece's home at 43 Gower Road in New Canaan, Connecticut.

On May 23, Signe attended the commencement exercises at the State University of New York at Buffalo by special invitation. She was there to receive the University Citation for "outstanding achievement in the field of physical rehabilitation as a pioneer in clinical investigation and an outstanding teacher." The idea of recognizing Signe came from Kathy Sawner with the support of J. Warren Perry, Dean of the School of Health Related Professions. Signe spent the weekend with Kathy. The busy two days included a dinner hosted by Kathy and Dean Perry honoring Signe with a champagne reception after the graduation ceremonies.

In his preamble to the presentation, University President Robert Keller indicated, " . . . the citation (was) the highest award that the State University of New York, on all of its campuses, (could) confer upon an individual. These citations, equivalent to the Honorary Doctorates conferred by many institutions, must be approved not only by the conferring institution, but by the Board of Trustees in Albany." He went on to describe Signe's early professional education and her teaching role at New York University and at the College of Physicians and Surgeons of Columbia University, as well as her association with Stanford and her services as a Fulbright lecturer in Greece. The President continued:

> She has been a pioneer in the development of improved techniques and approaches to physical rehabilitation. In an era when therapy techniques were derived from empiricism, the recipient pioneered the concept of 'inquiring clinician.' Her inquiry took her through years of observation, literature search, of failure and success in patient treatment. She demonstrated the courage of her convictions by publishing the results of her work, thereby challenging all allied health professionals to document their treatment methods. She has earned the respect and admiration of health practitioners and educators throughout the country.

While the president read the official University Citation, Signe was asked to join him at the podium. The citation stated:

> Signe Brunnstrom . . . having dedicated forty-five years of your life to the advancement of physical rehabilitation in America, you possess a singular ability to inspire all allied health professionals to integrate their knowledge and clinical skills for the betterment of patient care. At the heart of all of your professional endeavors has been an ever-present recognition of patients as persons. Although your own profession is physical therapy, you have constantly perceived that no allied health profession can accomplish its purpose in isolation. Your dream of well-defined concertation among health professions, which is also a goal of the School of Health Related Professions, is realized in your teaching achievements and your scholarly writings. As a frequent contributor to literature, your many publications have appeared in the professional journals of physical therapy, occupational therapy, and physical medicine. Both of your books, *Clinical Kinesiology* and *Movement Therapy in Hemiplegia*, are fundamental to the libraries of physical therapists and occupational therapists in this and other countries. As a pioneer in clinical investigation, health professionals in many fields are indebted to you. Because of your outstanding leadership in patient care, the State University of New York at Buffalo is honored to present to you its University Citation.

Signe prized the most-attractive award encased in a blue leather folder. Upon her return to New Canaan, she wrote Kathy how much she enjoyed the weekend: "Kathy, I hope that you will understand how much I appreciate all you have done for me professionally and personally. Your hospitality was something very special and the time I spent with you is dear to my heart." Kathy's reaction was: "to think that I had done something for her professionally! All I did was recognize her. She never sought glory and was somewhat bashful when it came her way. Her glory was in helping others, not in being glorified. I loved her for that, as did a host of other people."

Kathy received a letter on June 12 from Signe, indicating she would soon be leaving for Sweden and would "therefore be unable to carry on my professional correspondence in the U.S.A. from now on." It was at that point that Kathy became Signe's U.S.A. correspondent for hemiplegia workshops and other "Brunnstrom related activities."

During the summer, Rebel became weak and unable to walk and quietly passed away. After Rebel died, Signe had little reason to stay in this country and was ready to leave for Sweden.

She wrote Ruth Dickinson, advising her how to grant permission to use materials from *Clinical Kinesiology*. In her response, Ruth told Signe that she had received two royalty checks. "The money," she wrote on October 9 "is in a separate bank fund and I hope we can use it from time to time to further physical therapy education." Signe's reaction to the fund came in a letter of October 20. She wrote Ruth, "How nice of you to collect royalties from F. A. Davis Company with the view of furthering PT education and to let me know about it." She also mentioned that she was "taking off for Sweden," and expected to stay there for good. She regretted not being able to see the PT faculty before she left and particularly sent "best wishes to Cal (Mary Callahan) and Althea (Jones)." Her final comments were, "You have all been such good company and very helpful to me in many respects which I greatly appreciated."

On October 22, Signe left for Sweden to temporarily stay with her sister in Lund until she could find a place of her own.

In mid-November, a letter was forwarded to Signe from Harold Martinson, Editor, Harper & Row. It stated that, "the International Department has advised us that Ishiyaku Shuppan, who has the Japanese rights to publish your book, expects to publish the Japanese translation around April 1974." Signe wrote Martinson that she "would remain in Sweden for an indefinite period of time." She also asked that a copy of the Japanese translation be sent to her "at my permanent address, Norrevang 12, S-240 17 Sodra Sandby, Sweden."

Signe did not remain idle for very long. She called Kerstin Lundbladh and said, "I am here and ready to begin my work." Since the previous visit, Kerstin had become Superintendent Physical Therapist. As such, she had the facilities to accommodate Signe's work at the hospital. Signe needed a work permit. Kerstin recalled, "To take up employment in Swedish public health care at the age of seventy-five is quite unthinkable, a fact that Signe had some difficulty accepting." However, Signe was welcomed and "given every amenity." With Kerstin's assistance, Signe again was in her favorite environment. "Her work had enormous impact and far-reaching consequences for Swedish physical therapy generally and particularly for the physical therapists of Lund and their training at the University," Kerstin indicated.

Signe wrote Kathy on December 8, and described the process of "getting settled in the old country." She wrote of the problems she had getting a work permit, which actually took three months and was a source of great annoyance to her.

In January, 1974, Signe worked in the University Hospital three days a week. She divided her time between the neurology and rehabilitation units, and according to Kerstin, "expected everything to stop upon her arrival. Although we had to continue our normal duties, we tried to arrange to be with her whenever possible." Kerstin remembers the time well:

> Our working day grew longer, but Signe's presence, her opinions and our discussions made the work stimulating and exciting and utterly worthwhile. Life in the clinic was enriched equally for the patients who loved her and called her Aunt Signe.
>
> When she was not at the hospital she was scouring the University library for material which we could analyze at seminars she held at her home, some ten kilometers outside of Lund. She treated Saturday and Sunday and didn't seem to appreciate that we all had families demanding our attention at weekends at least.

> Her dedication was infectious and despite the extra work created, none of us regretted a single minute of the time spent with her.
>
> Life continued in this way for a year. Signe was tireless and often rang me when she had something interesting or when she had an idea she wanted to discuss. She would say, "I hope you're not doing anything in particular on Saturday. Do come and see me and let's talk." I am grateful to have been one of her discussion partners.

At the same time, Signe was planning a workshop on movement therapy in hemiplegia for therapists from all parts of Sweden.

Again in a letter of March 1974 to Kathy, Signe wrote:

> My responsibilities at Lund's Hospital have rapidly increased and lecture-demonstrations for the students at the PT school have been added. The audience has been enthusiastic. It took me considerable time to learn the correct Swedish words and occasionally I still have to use English expressions. My Swedish is improving and soon you might find Swedish words in my letters to you.
>
> At the present time I am turning down out-of-town engagements; it would be too strenuous while I am concentrating on training five group instructors for a workshop.

Kerstin realized Signe's goal was to arrange a course in the assessment and treatment of hemiplegic patients. "She probably kept her plans to herself until she could be certain of being able to train us as qualified assistants."

The winter months in Lund were cold, snowy, rainy, and windy and with much fog. Signe wrote: "now Spring is approaching and we occasionally have sunny days. My lawn is growing, snowdrops and crocus are out and buds are swelling." Obviously, she still found time to enjoy her surroundings and nature.

Always one to plan ahead, Signe prepared her last testament on May 6, 1974. As to funeral arrangements, Signe wished to be cremated, "the urn containing the ashes can be put in the Brunnstrom family grave in the New Cemetery in Helsingborg, Quarter B, Number 473-474."

A very special honor and recognition was given to Signe on May 18. The "Legitimerade Sjukgymnasters Riksforbund," the Swedish Association for Registered Physical Therapists, made her an honorary member. She was named the recipient of a certificate "for prominent contributions towards the Union of Physical Therapists," by the President, Greta Sifvert, at the Association's conference. Signe wrote a note of appreciation which stated:

> With gratitude I have received the beautiful document, showing that I have been chosen to honorary membership of LSR. In connection with the national conference for Swedish physical therapists in Linkoping, 1974, Kerstin Lundbladh presented it to me in the presence of a great number of physical therapists. Many thanks.

In June, Signe was able to conduct the special course through Lund University. Kerstin and her staff often wondered and asked each other what it was that kept Signe going. Part of the answer came in teaching the course. It was a great success, and according to Kerstin's observations: "it put Signe under tremendous strain, and when it was finished she was exhausted. She realized her ambition to share her knowledge of the improvement potential for hemiplegic patients, which was one of her principal reasons for returning to Sweden. Her commitment to the hemiplegic patient was complete."

In a letter of July 5, 1974, to Barbara White, then Assistant Editor of the APTA's *Journal of Physical Therapy*, Signe approved some mention of her return to Sweden to be published in the Journal. However, she made a point that her return was "not in order to continue my retirement." She indicated that she knew from an earlier trip to Lund, when she gave a lecture-demonstration on rehabilitation, that the medical and PT staff "wanted me to come back and I knew they had worthwhile work for me in mind." In the letter, Signe wrote: "I am struggling to learn the correct expressions and medical terms in Swedish and am slowly improving. From my present address, I am driving to work in Lund two to three days a week and the trip takes only fifteen to twenty minutes. It feels good to come home to my own house and garden where I grow mostly flowers, but also tomatoes. I never liked city living."

Barbara also needed a photo. Signe wrote, "I have no such picture, but possibly, my colleague and good friend Kathy Sawner may be able to get hold of one taken in Buffalo when I received a University Citation about a year ago, if a picture appears essential?"

Through her association with Signe at Lund, Kerstin realized that Signe faced many practical problems, which robbed her of the energy needed to adjust to the changes in Swedish society. "As long as she could concentrate on physical therapy," Kerstin wrote, "she could survive, and she demonstrated an impressive clarity of thought."

Signe still received mail at Columbia and Ruth saw to it that important letters were forwarded. One such letter of July 17, was from William D. Winston, Medical Editor of Yearbook Medical Publishers in Chicago. He raised the possibility of Signe writing a "concise, practical manual on kinesiology." Signe responded to that suggestion in a letter of August 10, in which she suggested, "it would first be necessary to find out for what category of professional students and instructors the manual is intended." She also wrote, "from your letter I cannot deduce whether or not you are aware of my book 'Clinical Kinesiology' which is directed mainly to physical therapists and other medical personnel. The book is now in its 3rd edition (1972), an edition that was prepared by Ruth Dickinson of Columbia University." Rather than getting herself involved with Yearbook Publishers, Signe suggested that Mr. Winston save "time-consuming correspondence across the Atlantic Ocean by contacting Ruth, who could "probably give good advice."

Signc also mentioned that, "Professor Dickinson would be an excellent person to write a brief, concise manual on Kinesiology if there is a need for such a manual." A handwritten comment on the carbon copy sent to Ruth indicated how much Signe missed her friends, "I often wish I could have a chat with Cal, you and Althea. No I can only say 'hello' to all of you, and thanks for forwarding letters to me."

When the article about Signe's return to Sweden appeared in the *Journal of Physical Therapy*, one therapist, Charlotte Weithem wrote Signe the following "(Dec. 9, 1974)":

> Dear Miss Brunnstrom:
>
> In the American Physical Therapy journal I read that you left the USA. You probably do not remember me, I met you years ago in the Rusk Institute. I shall never forget your fascinating and stimulating techniques and am very grateful to you that you allowed me to attend your classes. Though I never met you again, I wanted you to know that I am really sorry you left us. The best of luck in 1975 and every year.

As busy as Signe was in Sweden, she did not let that letter go unanswered. She responded:

> I appreciate getting your letter of December 9. Of course I remember you very well and am glad if anything you picked up at Rusk's place has benefited some patients of yours, whether amputees, hemi-patients or others. I have been busy at the Rehab Clinic in Lund, mainly with hemiplegic patients, and busy at home writing a compendium (in Swedish) needed for a workshop on hemiplegia for Swedish PT's from various parts of Sweden. It was not an easy job. Have had success as well as disappointments and frustrations, but that I guess is life. Best wishes for health and happiness.
>
> As ever
> Signe

In mid-December, 1974, I as Chairman of the Department of Physical Therapy at the State University of New York at Stony Brook, corresponded with Signe. The letter came as a result of a decision (made by the Chairman with faculty members Michael Helland, Clifton S. Mereday, Barbara Silvestri, and staff, Gloria Mitchell) to invite Signe to Long Island and offer a week-long continuing education workshop and a weekend seminar. The Long Island District of the APTA would be a co-sponsor. Signe agreed to the arrangements. Several of her colleagues were also invited to assist her in the workshop, including Kathy Sawner, Jeanne LaVigne, Mary Ann Suda and Susan Scheer. They all accepted the invitation. Following another letter requesting a recent photo, Signe wrote me on February 27, 1975, expressing her concern for all the work that had to be done to arrange a workshop:

> Here is a snapshot of me taken in 1973. It is the only one that I possess. Hope it serves the purpose you have in mind. Glad to hear that arrangements for the symposium continue—it must require a great deal of work for you.

Signe returned to Connecticut late in May, 1975. Ruth Dickinson drove her to Stony Brook for the weekend conference of June 6–7. The sessions were held in the south campus of the university in a large room. The weekend seminar was attended by 144 therapists and 32 students. During her presentations, Signe often had a momentary lapse of memory. She occasionally seemed confused and unable to complete a statement. Kathy Sawner caught every nuance and often stepped in to continue the discussion. Signe was not in control of her presentation.

The workshop was held at the Oak Hollow Nursing Center and was limited to 16 therapists. Here again, Signe was unable to maintain control of her demonstrations. The program evaluations were all highly positive. However, it was obvious to many of the therapists that they were witnesses to what would be the last major presentation on hemiplegia presented by Signe Brunnstrom.

A reception and banquet to honor Signe was held at the Three Village Inn in Stony Brook one evening after the seminar. Signe was the center of attraction. She was presented with an engraved watch and flowers. The "master therapist" again demonstrated her humility in limiting her response, but those in attendance warmly applauded her for the years of service to the profession. It was an emotional evening for all!

For her role in the two programs, Signe was paid $1,264, which included an honorarium, local travel and accommodations. Her round-trip airfare to Sweden was paid separately. In a true demonstration of her concern for students, Signe donated several hundred dollars to the Stony Brook and the Buffalo PT program "for use of the students as might be necessary." Buffalo established a clinical education scholarship/loan fund for exceptional students who wished to participate in clinical activities oriented towards clinical research. Stony Brook set the funds aside to assist students in need of immediate short-term loans to help them overcome a financial problem. Signe's charitable gesture continues to benefit students today, as it has done over the past years.

Upon her return to Sweden, Signe was not well, but she continued working with Kerstin Lundbladh on a hemiplegia publication. (The co-authored 80-page booklet, entitled *Hemiplegi—introduktion till rorelsebehandling*, was published in Sweden in September, 1976.) Kerstin recalled that when Signe worked at the hospital and the university: "I felt as if she was in a hurry in order to teach Swedish P.T.s. Signe and I talked a lot about many things, but she did not talk much about herself, and I never asked. Her mind was occupied by physical therapy . . . " Kerstin suggested: "After fifty years abroad, it was not easy to feel at home in Sweden, and she often spoke of the United States as her home. She used to express her pride and joy in her American citizenship."

By late Autumn, Signe showed increasing difficulty in orienting herself to time and space. It became questionable if she could live alone. In November, 1975, Signe was seen at the University Hospital in Lund. After a thorough examination, she was diagnosed as having a duodenal ulcer. Surgery was recommended, but Signe wanted to return to the states and have surgery at Norwalk Hospital in Connecticut. Her niece, Elsa, came to Lund to take her back to the states. When Signe was admitted to Norwalk Hospital in late November, it was determined that she had a five-year history of stomach problems which had been treated conservatively with oral medications. At Norwalk, a subtotal gastrectomy was performed, and Signe was discharged just before Christmas "(December 23,)" to Elsa's home in New Canaan. Elsa Diehl was the only relative in the states that Signe could turn to. She took on a great responsibility in caring for her aunt. Signe's mental and physical health deteriorated rapidly. It soon became evident that Elsa was unable to offer Signe adequate care in her home. The decision was made to place Signe in the Waveny Care Center, and she entered the facility on January 28, 1976 at 3:45. Signe was a very difficult patient and did not adjust to the center. She became more confused and debilitated. On April 21, she was admitted to a larger facility, the Darien Convalescent Center.

In November, 1983, at the annual meeting of the American Society of Allied Health Professions, held in Philadelphia, I inquired about Signe in a conversation with Kathy Sawner. Kathy indicated she was in a nursing home. It was obvious that it was difficult for Kathy to talk about Signe's mental and physical condition. A few days later, I wrote Elsa Diehl, inquiring about Signe's health. Her response indicated the gravity of the situation:

> Unfortunately she is living in the Darien Convalescent Center and has done so for the last eight years. There she gets moved from her bed to a chair and back again. She can do nothing for herself and does not speak. I go there once a week to talk to her and feed her. I keep doing it but don't know if she even knows who I am. I hope that sometimes she remembers a song, a poem, or a person that I mention. It is sad and strange and you feel helpless. She clings to "life" and

> I cling to a hope that she is not suffering and maybe there is something, some meaning I don't understand.

With Elsa Diehl's encouragement, the decision to write Signe's biography was made. Thanks to Elsa's cooperation, access was granted to all of Signe's papers. Many documents and photographs were made available. A chronological outline of Signe's life and work was prepared. Individual letters to many of Signe's professional colleagues, her friends and former students brought an out-pouring of anecdotes and comments. All have been integrated into the total biography.

In December, 1985, I arranged to travel to Sweden to meet with Signe's two sisters. In the Stockhlom area, I received complete cooperation from Ingegerd Brunnstrom Westerlund. Then I flew to Lund in southern Sweden to visit Signe's older sister, Elsa Brunnstrom Diehl. While in Lund, I also met with Signe's dear friend, Kerstin Lundbladh.

As work on the biographical manuscript progressed, correspondence with Ms. Phyllis Quinn, APTA's Coordinator of Information Services and the Archives of Physical Therapy, resulted in another approach to promoting the history of physical therapy. I submitted an abstract for a "Brunnstrom" poster session for the Annual Conference of the American Physical Therapy Association, to be held in Chicago, June 8–12, 1986. Frank Allender, APTA's Director of Program Development, recommended a very special handling of the poster session. Instead of remaining on view for only one day, the Brunnstrom pictorial history was shown for three consecutive days. The poster, "4 feet x 16 feet", consisted of family and childhood photographs, educational documents, military papers, special manuscripts, professional notes and personal items, all tracing 87 years of Signe Brunnstrom's life and professional activities.

The poster session was well received. Carol M. Davis, Ed.D., of Boston University wrote on October 6, 1986:

> Just wanted to thank you for your pictorial history of Signe Brunnstrom. I value, so much, the contribution of the physical therapists who came before us to carve out the strong foundations upon which we now grow to

greater understanding and relevance in health care intervention and prevention. You have captured the growth and personhood of such a significant contributor to physical therapy. Her life was so rich and valuable, her legacy lives on in her work and life, captured so eloquently by your camera and your heart. Thank you, Jay, for caring so much about us to contribute this for us. We are all better for it.

How should Signe Brunnstrom be remembered? People in rehabilitation are aware of her professional work, but so few people actually knew the personal side of Signe Brunnstrom. Despite all of the attention and acclaim she received for her contributions, she was a lonely person who lived to work. She also was an author, clinician, researcher, educator, naturalist, builder, humanitarian and friend. Her presence on the good earth touched many people. What legacy did she leave and how do you summarize her life's contributions? Perhaps such a summary should be left to some of Signe's close professional associates:

Geneva Johnson of Houston, Texas, wrote:

> The approach she demonstrated to patient care was scientific but caring. She made no unsupported claims for the results she achieved in her work with patients. No cult developed around her approach to patient care. She discouraged that by urging her colleagues to investigate the alternative approaches available. She was a pioneer in our field; a person of great intellect, integrity, and character; a major contributor to our literature; and an exceptional physical therapy clinician.

From Jack Hofkosh of New York City:

> To see her ideas and practices come to fruition must have been heart-warming for Signe. Thank you Signe for all your guidance, encouragement and patience for over 30 years of my practice as a physical therapist. You taught me, not only skills in managing the amputee, and the brain- damaged, but inquisitiveness, toler-

ance and above all to seek the highest level to which I could attain.

From G. Gordon Williamson of Edison, New Jersey:

Upon reflection there is one overriding reason why this remarkable individual has influenced my personal and professional life so strongly. Signe is the very model of a scholarly clinician. She would focus on a major clinical issue and pursue it diligently for years. She would study the area extensively, integrate the reading into her practice, experiment and discover, and then publish her findings. There was a conscious link of theory, practice and professional writing throughout her long career. She demonstrated this recurring cycle in her work in the rehabilitation of patients with amputations and cerebral vascular accidents as well as her contribution to clinical kinesiology. Signe paid a price for her commitment to scholarly practice. She worked at a furious pace and at times subsisted on part-time employment in order to have time for library research and study. Consequently she lived quite frugally. Her values were clearly committed to using intellectual inquiry for practical purposes in order to benefit her patients. As a result the entire field of rehabilitation has been enriched. For such a gift we can all be grateful.

From Mary Callahan of New York City:

The name Signe Brunnstrom brings forth a myriad of experiences and impressions. To me, she represents a major influence in the development of physical therapy as a science . . . (and as) an art. Signe had many interests;, a devotion to teaching and to young people . . . (she was) a lover of animals (especially dogs), a good cook, a lover of nature and home (her gardens, her property). It did not phase her to mow the lawn, chop wood or tackle a tree . . . a versatile person, a perfectionist.

From Betty Canan in Birmingham, Alabama:

How fortunate we are that she (immigrated) to the United States. Think of the void we would have in our profession without her legacy of knowledge, special skills, and textbooks.

Samuel Feitelberg of Burlington, Vermont, wrote:

The use of her hands was astounding as she touched and guided patients, one moment tapping, the next moment pulling and pushing. She appeared like a photographer posing the client for that special portrait, when in reality she was bringing forward a movement to be generated by the patient. What satisfaction and pure joy when they moved something as if she directed it to happen. Her techniques were not hocus-pocus but her personal touch was that of healing hands.

From L. Don Lehmkuhl, Houston, Texas,:

She has truly been one of the great clinicians, clinical researchers and educators of our profession. The high degree of intellectual curiosity she possessed, coupled with acute powers of observation and deductive reasoning led her to keep copious notes on the natural history of recovery from damage to the nervous system. To make the pertinent findings of researchers available to her students and other clinicians, Signe translated the articles and prepared English summaries of them. She was among the first physical therapists to formulate a protocol for assessing and treating neurological disorders based on her understandings of neurophysiological mechanisms.

Stuart MacRoberts of Savannah, Georgia, wrote:

I am proud to have had the opportunity to know Signe, and wish everyone could be as fortunate. She was very humble, and yet she was a leader in her field. She looked for ways to improve care of people. Her work with amputees during WWII was of great benefit to us all. And she used some of her original thoughts on amputee care in the stroke rehab programs, I don't believe she ever stopped looking for new and improved ways of doing things. She was open to suggestions and listened to everyone no matter what their knowledge. If the suggestions were appropriate, she used them to improve her techniques.

I never heard Signe put anyone down. She maintained that her philosophy of treatment was only one way, and if her way did not work, then she encouraged you to try something else. There is no one way of treatment, but many possible ways. You observe what works for that particular person and go with it. If after a while the one way is not effective any longer, then rethink the problem, do clinical observation, try different techniques, be open for improvement. Signe's philosophy was "you do what will help the patient." Perhaps that concept has had the greatest influence on me.

From Kerstin Lundbladh, Lund, Sweden:

The one year Signe Brunnstrom was actively involved in physical therapy in Sweden has played a significant part in its development. As a result of her searching and critical attitude, Signe has to a high degree contributed to the problem-orientation that characterizes the direction of physical therapy in Sweden today. As elsewhere methods had become, to a greater or lesser extent, the ends instead of the means. Whilst teaching her individual approach she encouraged us to experiment. "It does not matter what you are doing as long as you know what you want and the patient responds." Such freedom of action was new to many Swedish physical therapists.

It is my opinion that Signe Brunnstrom's work in Lund stressed the importance of studied functional analysis as a basis for a more productive application of personal physical therapy skills. Swedish physical therapy is greatly indebted to Signe Brunnstrom.

From Harold E. Potts of Northford, Connecticut:

Signe Brunnstrom is remembered as a sincere and concerned friend, a dynamic and inspiring teacher and a highly respected clinician; a spirited and loveable personality. When in her presence one could not resist feeling a deep sense of respect for the Lady. Signe's hallmark was her analytic and discerning mind. As a clinician, her ability to visually dissect the human structure, to palpate and describe the actions of muscles and joints relative to normal and abnormal movement was uncanny.

Signe Brunnstrom made the practice of physical therapy truly an excitement.

From Kathy Sawner of Buffalo, New York:

She once told me she never had a full-time job because a physical therapist could not both work full time and learn all that was necessary to good performance. One could learn a lot from Signe, and not just about stroke patients and amputees. She delighted in getting to know people, even though she was shy and hated to be fussed over. There was so much to be learned from Signe and I shall be eternally grateful for the privilege of knowing her. She touched and enriched countless lives through her dedication to physical therapy and the patients entrusted to our care. Her involvement with hemiplegia began after the polio epidemic and was really a response to the frustration she encountered among therapists on her wide-spread travels around the country. Their orientation to management of polio patients was not readily transferable to patients with CNS disorders. Therapists didn't feel good about what they were doing with stroke patients and the patients weren't getting better, so Signe became the champion of both. Perhaps that is her legacy: to recognize that things could be better and to endeavor to make them so.

On Sunday morning, February 21, 1988, after a lengthy illness, Signe Brunnstrom died at the age of 90. She had been a resident of the Darien Convalescent Center in Darien, Connecticut since April, 1976.

As requested in her will, cremation took place with burial planned for the family plot in Helsingborg, Sweden.

Signe's relatives asked for Kerstin's opinion as to what should be done with all of the material. Should Signe's collected papers be left in Lund or sent back to the United States?

"I told them that as I learned to know Signe," Kerstin indicated, "I understood that she was very proud to be an American citizen. She told me that the U.S. government and American physical therapists appreciated her work more so than in any country." Kerstin also recognized that Signe lived most of her life in the United States and did her greatest work here. Kerstin wrote, "That is why I am quite sure Signe's own will would be that all the material belongs in the United States."

I was given the honor to be responsible for the disposition of the Brunnstrom papers. " 'I have full confidence in your decisions about this,'' wrote Ms. Lundbladh.

In May 1989, I received six boxes from the University of Lund and one large box from Elsa Diehl. Contents included hand-written notes, hundreds of photographs used by Signe in her publications, copies of correspondence, reports of projects, official documents and reprints of her articles.

In expectation that the collection will be of interest to physical therapists in the future, the Brunnstrom papers will be placed in the Archives of Physical Therapy maintained by the American Physical Therapy Association in Alexandria, Virginia.

Appendix I

Signe Brunnstrom's Professional Contributions

Books and Films

Books

Leg Amputee: Preprosthetic Training. Rehabilitation Series No. 3.(Co-author, D. Kerr). West Orange, New Jersey: The Kessler Institute for Rehabilitation, 1951. Illus., 44 pp.

Training of the Lower Extremity Amputee. (Co-author, D. Kerr). Springfield. IL: Charles C Thomas, 1956. Illus., 272 pp.

Clinical Kinesiology. Philadelphia: F.A. Davis Company, 1962. Illus., 339 pp. Second Printing, 1966.

Clinical Kinesiology. Second Edition, 1966. Second Printing, March 1967. Third Printing, November 1968. Fourth Printing, November 1970.

Movement Therapy in Hemiplegia: A Neurophysiological Approach. New York: Harper and Row, Publishers, 1970. Illus., 192 pp.

Clinical Kinesiology. Third Edition, Revision by Ruth Dickinson. Philadelphia: F.A. Davis Co., 1972. Second Printing, 1973. Third Printing, 1973.

Movement Therapy in Hemiplegia. Japanese Edition, Tokio: Ishiyaku Shuppan, Publisher, 1974.

Hemiplegia—Introduktion Till Rorelsebehandling Swedish language edition with Kerstin Lundbladh. Lund, Sweden: Studentlitteratur, 80 pp. 1977.

Movement Therapy in Hemiplegia. Spanish Edition, Revision by Maria Victoria Carbo De Valls. Barcelona, Spain. Editorial JIMS, 1977.

Movement Therapy in Hemiplegia. Second printing in Spanish, 1979.

Brunnstroms's Clinical Kinesiology. L. Don Lehmkuhl & Laura K.Smith, Editors. Philadelphia: F.A. Davis, Publishers, Philadelphia, 453 pp. 1983.

Chapters in Books

"The Lower Extremity Amputee, Chapter XIX", *Physical Medicine in General Practice*. Edited by Bierman and Licht, New York: Paul B. Hoeber, 1952.

"Anatomical and Physiological Considerations in the Clinical Application of Lower-Extremity Prosthetics. Chapter 9" *Orthopedic Appliances Atlas*, Vol. 2, Ann Arbor, MI.: J. W. Edwards, Ed.. American Academy of Orthopedic Surgeons. 1960.

Films

Aftercare of Leg Amputations. Prepared at U.S. Naval Hospital, Mare Island, CA., 1945-46. 16mm., silent, color. Running time: one hour.

Peripheral Nerve Injuries. (2 films) Prepared at U.S. Naval Hospital Mare Island, CA., 1945-46. 16mm., silent, color. Running time: 20 min.

Suction Socket Amputee Training. Prepared at the Prosthetic and Testing Laboratory of the Veterans Administration, New York, N.Y., under the auspices of the Advisory Committee on Artificial Limbs of the National Research Council, 1948. 16mm., silent, black and white. Running time: about 20 min.

Training of the Arm in Adult Patients with Hemiplegia. Prepared at the Institute of Physical Medicine and Rehabilitation, New York University-Bellevue Medical Center, 1955. 16mm., silent, black and white. Running time: about 30 min.

Neurophysiologic Influences in the Restoration of Function in Adult Patients with Hemiplegia. (In cooperation with Glenn C.Reynolds, M.D.) Prepared at the Institute of Physical Medicine and Rehabilitation, New York University-Bellevue Medical Center, 1957. 16mm sound, color. Running time: 30 min.

Appendix II

Articles by Signe Brunnstrom

1. "Faulty Weight Bearing: With Special Reference to Position of Thigh and Foot." *The Physiother. Rev.*, Vol. 15, No.3, 1935.
2. "The Changing Conception of Posture: Methods of Dealing with Faulty Posture." *The Physiother. Rev.*, Vol. 20, No. 2, 1940.
3. "Muscle Group Testing." *The Physiother. Rev.*, Vol. 21, No. 1, 1941.
4. "Muscle Testing Around the Shoulder Girdle: A Study of the Function of Shoulderblade Fixators in Seventeen Cases of Shoulder Paralysis." *J. Bone & Joint Surg.*, 23:263–272, 1941.
5. "Some Observations of Muscle Function: With Special Reference to Pluriarticular Muscles." *The Physiother. Rev.*, Vol. 22, No. 2, 1942.
6. "Physical Therapy in the Aftercare of Amputations of the Lower Extremity." *U.S. Naval Medical Bulletin*, 43:634–644, 1944.
7. "Comparative Strength of Muscles with Similar Function: A Study of Peripheral Nerve Injuries of the Upper Extremity." *The Physiother. Rev.*, Vol. 26, No. 2, 1946.

8. "Walking Training of the Amputee: Some Biomechanical Considerations." *The Physiother. Rev.*, Vol. 27, No.3, 1947.
9. "Suction Socket Amputee Training." *The Orthop. Appliance & Limb Manuf. Assoc. Journal*, Autumn 1948.
10. "Amputee Training in Greece". *The Phys. Ther. Rev.*, 31:419–426, 1951. (This article was translated into German by Prof. Thomson, and appeared in Orthopedie-Technik, Vol. 4, No. 7, July 1952.)
11. "Heltung," Chap. III of *Korperstellung* (Body Posture) by Rudolph Magnus, translated and abstracted by S. Brunnstrom: *Phys. Ther. Rev.*, Vol. 33, No. 6, June 1953.
12. "Head Posture and Muscle Tone, Clinical Observations" A. Simons, translated and abstracted by S. Brunnstrom: *Phys. Ther. Rev.*, Vol. 33, No. 8, August 1953.
13. "Center-of-Gravity Line in Relation to Ankle Joint in Erect Standing: Application to Posture Training and to Artificial Legs." *Phys. Ther. Rev.*, 34:109–115, 1954.
14. "Associated Reactions of the Upper Extremity in Adult Patients with Hemiplegia: An Approach to Training." *Phys. Ther. Rev.*, 36:225–236, 1956.
15. "Methods Used to Elicit, Reinforce and Coordinate Muscular Responses in Upper Motor Neuron Lesions." *APTA-OVR Institute Papers*, Part III, 1956. Adult Patients with Hemiplegia, pp. 100–114.
16. "The Use of Associated Reaction Patterns in the Training of Adult Patients with Hemiplegia." *Proceedings, Second Congress World Confederation for Physical Therapy*, pp. 55–61, 1956. Published by the Am. Phys. Ther. Assoc., 1790 Broadway, New York, NY.
17. "Preliminary Report on Neuromuscular Function Testing of the Upper Extremity in Adult Hemiplegic Patients." Co-authors: G. Reynolds and N. Thompson: *Arch. Phys. Med.*, 39:303–310, 1958.
18. "Problems of Sensorimotor Learning in the Evaluation and Treatment of the Adult Hemiplegic Patient." G. Reynolds co-author. *Rehab. Liter.*, 20:163–171, 1959.

19. "Motor Behavior of Adult Hemiplegic Patients: Hints for Training." *Am. J. Occup. Ther.*, 15:6–12, 1961.
20. "Recording Gait Patterns of Adult Hemiplegic Patients." *J. Amer. Phys. Ther. Assoc.*, 44:11–18, 1964.
21. "Walking Preparation for Adult Patients with Hemiplegia." *J. Amer. Phys. Ther. Assoc.*, 45:17–29, 1965.
22. "Motor Testing Procedures in Hemiplegia: Based on Sequential Recovery Stages." Accepted for publication in J. Amer. Phy. Ther. Assoc., 1966. (April Issue)

Research Reports

Participation in Report to National Research Council, Committee on Artificial Limbs, in *Fundamental Studies of Human Locomotion and Other Information Relating to Design of Artificial Limbs*. University of California, Berkeley, 1947.

Section 10, Amputee Training, in *Investigations With Respect to Design, Construction and Evaluation of Prosthetic Devices* Vol. 2, Research Division, College of Engineering, New York University. Report to Office of Naval Research, Special Devices Center, Sands Point, L.I., NY, 1948.

Report on the Study of Neurophysiologic Reactions Facilitating Recovery Following Hemiplegia. Institute of Physical Medicine and Rehabilitation, New York University-Bellevue Medical Center, 1957. Co-investigator, G. Reynolds, M.D.

Appendix III

Brunnstrom Information Contacts

Dr. Anthony Ackerman, Carmel, NY
William Ammerman, Athens, Greece
Harry Bates, Carmel, NY
Alice Berg, P.T., Waukesha, WI
Mary Binderman, Rockville, MD
Lucy Blair, Peterborough, NH (Deceased)
Ellen Blodgett, P.T., Ft. Montgomery, NY
Bonnie Blossom, P.T., Atlanta, GA
William Brooks, P.T., Syosset, NY (Deceased)
Margaret M. Brown, St. Petersburg, FL
Mary Eleanor Brown, P.T., Morro Bay, CA
Dean Robert Burnham, Washington Square, NY
Mary Callahan, P.T., NY, NY
Betty Canan, P.T., Pelham, AL
Phillip Carson, Uniondale, NY
Paul Collura, DDS, Carmel, NY
Virginia Consiglio, P.T., NY, NY
Robert H. Craven, Philadelphia, PA.
Lucille Daniels, P.T., Belmont, CA
Carol Davis, Ed.D., P.T., Boston, MA
Ruby Decker, P.T., Galveston, TX

Anthony DeRosa, P.T., Hartsdale, NY
Ruth Dickinson, P.T., Ft. Lee, NJ
Elsa Diehl, Westport, CT
Elsa Brunnstrom Diehl, Lund, Sweden
Harry Doppelt, P.T., Cold Spring, NY
Editorial JIMS, Barcelona 6, Spain
Betty Edwards, P.T., Bellair Bluffs, FL
Mildred Elson, P.T., (Deceased), Boynton Beach, FL
Peter English, NY, NY
Paul S. Entmacher, M.D., NY, NY
Emily "Sue" Fairbanks, P.T., Bradenton, FL
Sam Feitelberg, P.T., Burlington, VT
Mary Flickinger, P.T., Hinsdale, IL
Marie Louise Franciscus, O.T.R., North Fort Meyers, FL
James J. Garibaldi, Rockville, MD
Louis Greenwald, P.T., Dubuque, IA
Bud Haley, P.T., Modesto, CA
Michael M. Helland, P.T., Ormond Beach, FL
James Herrington, P.T., Greensburg, PA
Helen Hickey, P.T., Waltham, MA
Susanne Hirt, P.T., Richmond, VA
Helen Hislop, Ph.D., P.T., Downey, CA
Jack Hofkosh, NY, NY
Marjorie Ionta, P.T., Weymouth, MA
George Jessup, P.T., Panama City, FL
Geneva Johnson, Ph.D., P.T., Houston, TX
Althea Jones, P.T., Franklin Lakes, NJ
Herbert Jones, P.T., North Miami, FL
Helen Kaiser, P.T., (Deceased), Durham, NC
Donald Kerr, Ruston, LA
Bruce Kodish, P.T., NY, NY
Gary Krasilovsky, P.T., Westport, CT
Francoise Lamote, PT-OT, Ajaccio, France
Jeanne LaVigne, P.T., Yorktown Heights, NY
L. Don Lehmkuhl, Ph.D.,P.T., Houston, TX
Colonel Matts Liljegren, Stockholm, Sweden
Georgia Loescher, P.T., Kansas City, MO
Kerstin Lundbladh, P.T., Lund, Sweden
Stuart MacRoberts, P.T., Savannah, GA

Harvey Margolin, P.T., Carmel, NY
Muriel Mahon, Ave., Flushing, NY
Medical Dept., Harper & Row Publishers NY, NY
Clifton S. Mereday, Ph.D., P.T. Hauppauge, NY
Eugene Michels, Ph.D., P.T., College Park, MD
David Miller, Baltimore, MD
Joan Mohr, P.T., Cresskill, NJ
Margaret Moore, Ph.D., P.T., Holly Ridge, NC
Marian Oliva NY, NY
Lorraine Paulson, P.T., Denver, CO
Joseph Peleso, Jr., Carmel, NY
Alice and William Polatnick, St. James, NY
Harold E. Potts, P.T., Northford, CT
Elfriede Prins, P.T., Gresham, OR
Phyllis Quinn, Alexandria, VA
Kathy Romenski, P.T., Scranton, PA
Fred Rutan, P.T., (Deceased), Alburquerque, NM
Kathryn Sawner, P.T., Buffalo, NY
Barbara Schad, P.T., NY, NY
Martha Schnebly, O.T.R., Ph.D. Detroit, MI
Sarah Semans, P.T., Palo Alto, CA
Gladys Semeryan, Washington, DC
Virginia Shaw, NY, NY
Barbara Silvestri, P.T., Valley Stream, NY
William Sippel, Ph.D., Albany, NY
Barb Skewes, Alexandria, VA
Arthur Spell, P.T., Stratford, NJ
Floyd Spurgeon, P.T., Alliance, OH
Lucy Gore Stead, O.T.R., Vancouver, B.C. Canada
Gerald Stern, P.T., Baldwin, NY
John R. Steves, Cleveland Hts, OH
Fran Tappan, Ed.D., P.T., Storrs, CT
Robert Teckemeyer, P.T., Fort Royal, VA
Payne Thomas, Springfield, IL
Major Mary J. Torp, P.T., USA-Ret, Del City, OK
Anna Urband, Washington DC
Charles Verderese, Carmel, NY
Veterans Affairs, Salt Lake City, UT
Dorothy Voss, P.T., Weymouth, MA

L.S. Watts, Mare Island, CA
Ingegerd Brunnstrom Westerlund, Lund, Sweden
G. Gordon Williamson, Ph.D., O.T.R., Edison, NJ
Catherine Worthingham, Ph.D., P.T., Belmont, CA
Natalie Zucker, Santa Fe Springs, CA

Appendix IV

Award Named in Honor of Signe Brunnstrom

On August 11, 1987, I wrote Lydia Wingate, Ph.D., President of the New York Chapter of the American Physical Therapy Association, suggesting the Chapter Board take action to initiate an honor in recognition of Signe Brunnstrom for her valuable contributions to physical therapy. It was proposed that the chapter submit a resolution to the American Physical Therapy Association recommending that the recently established Award for Excellence in Clinical Teaching be named the Signe Brunnstrom Award for Excellence in Clinical Teaching.

Dr. Wingate presented the letter to the Chapter Board at the September, 1987 board meeting and a resolution was passed and forwarded to National.

At the November, 1987 APTA Board of Directors' meeting, under the leadership of President Jane Mathews, the board accepted the resolution. Signe Brunnstrom's name was attached to the award as of January, 1988.

The first presentation of the Signe Brunnstrom Award for Excellence in Clinical Teaching took place at the APTA's annual conference in Las Vegas on June 14, 1988. The recipient was Kathleen Menella, Director of the Department of

Therapies at Orthopaedic Hospital in Los Angeles. I was honored to make the presentation.